Advance Praise for
OPEN YOUR MOUTH!:
*How the Right Conversation with Your Dentist
Can Change Your Life*

Integrity, excellence, and patient-centered describe Drs. Christian Yaste and Joe Hufanda. *Open Your Mouth!* is worth your time and attention because Yaste and Hufanda have first opened their eyes and ears to the questions and anxieties of our dental needs and health. As you listen to their stories and absorb their experience you will discover that you are not alone in your concerns. Read, reflect, and step toward a better future with "your mouth" and "your life" together with Yaste and Hufanda.

BRYAN AALBORG, D. MIN.
Lead Pastor, Sharon Seventh-day Adventist Church
Charlotte, NC

I met Dr. Christian Yaste and Dr. Joe Hufanda at a business seminar several years ago. It was clear to me then, as it is now, that they're more than just dentists. Over time, I've watched them grow their families and their practice, seeing first-hand their commitment to the highest levels of compassion, conscientiousness, performance, and care in every aspect of their lives. Their professional work speaks volumes. This book is a commitment from Drs. Yaste and Hufanda to provide you with information that can change the direction of your life.

MICHAEL YORK
Author, speaker and CEO of Michael York
Mastermind Consulting, Inc.

Sometimes research surprises even the best of experts and that is what happened to me. For years I have been under the impression that people with bad teeth were a product of neglect and were not heeding their dentist's advice. It turns out that your genetics play a critical role in teeth and gum health, and often times there just isn't enough you can do to reverse that. Fortunately, there is help and there are answers. Dr. Yaste and Dr. Hufanda clear the air and dispel the myths that so many dental patients have been led to believe. The dentally challenged no longer have to carry a burden of shame. If you have lived through dental embarrassment, *Open Your Mouth!* is a must read.

LANE OSTROW J.D. , LL.M.
Founder of HonorOne, LLC and Executive Director
of the Global PTSI Foundation

For many years I was afraid of dentists. I feared the pain, discomfort, stress, and squirming in the dental chair with the sound of the drill digging into my molars. I hated the date of the next appointment, the day of the visit, sitting in the chair anticipating that moment when the drill hits a nerve and sends that shock of pain that I knew would happen again and again. As a patient of Drs. Yaste and Hufanda, I no longer have that experience. They have changed all that. Their goal in this book is to do the same for you, providing a blueprint for navigating and changing anything and everything negative connected with the dental visit.

JOHN PAUL GALLES
Publisher, *Charlotte Biz Magazine* & CLT.biz

Open Your Mouth! is an engaging, reader-friendly, passionate book about how two dentists—Drs. Christian Yaste and Joe Hufanda—long-time friends who practice their craft at Ballantyne Center for Dentistry, make dentistry work for practically everyone. The book especially targets the layperson that dreads going to the dentist. With understanding and compassion, they discuss what's new in dentistry, what's gone awry in dentistry, and how, through their holistic approach, they seek a life-time dental healthcare partnership with each of their patients. If you are one of those people who have painful memories of past dental experiences and would rather be kicked in the shins than go to a dentist, this book is for you.

ELEANOR GREEN BSN
President, Frederick Nursing Consultants;
Coauthor: *Clinical Practice Guidelines for the Adult*
Patient; Managing Quality: A Guide to Monitoring
and Evaluating Nursing Services; Managing Quality:
A Guide to System-Wide Performance Management
in Healthcare

While Joe and Christian wrote this book with the patient in mind, every dentist should read it. At its core, this body of work is about passion, caring, and love for the dental profession and the patients it serves – something every dentist who strives for joy in their professional career and success in their practice needs to be reminded of. The stories are heart-warming and the lessons are priceless, so whether you are a prospective patient or a dental professional, sit back and drink from this fountain of wisdom from two of the most gifted and successful dentists I've ever had the pleasure of knowing.

ANTHONY FECK, DMD
Sunrise Dental Solutions

This book will introduce you to the new world of dentistry and technology, a better world of less (or no!) pain and more possibilities. Corporate dentistry or private practice? Electric toothbrush or manual brush? Dental implants? Dr. Yaste and Dr. Hufanda will introduce you to many people and their circumstances, and you will learn that you are not alone. From tooth whitening to veneers, sedation dentistry to dental implants, plus cost and getting the most bang for your buck, it's all right here.

JOHN HANCOCK
WBT Radio Hall of Fame Recipient
WBT Radio Charlotte, NC

OPEN YOUR MOUTH!

OPEN YOUR MOUTH!

*How the Right Conversation
with Your Dentist
Can Change Your Life*

Dr. Christian Yaste and Dr. Joe Hufanda

NEW YORK

LONDON • NASHVILLE • MELBOURNE • VANCOUVER

OPEN YOUR MOUTH!

How the Right Conversation with Your Dentist Can Change Your Life

Published in New York, New York, by Morgan James Publishing. Morgan James is a trademark of Morgan James, LLC. www.MorganJamesPublishing.com

The Morgan James Speakers Group can bring authors to your live event. For more information or to book an event visit The Morgan James Speakers Group at www.TheMorganJamesSpeakersGroup.com.

ISBN 9781683506218 paperback
ISBN 9781683506225 eBook
Library of Congress Control Number: 2017909235

Cover Design by:
Megan Whitney
megan@creativeninjadesigns.com

Interior Design by:
Chris Treccani
www.3dogcreative.net

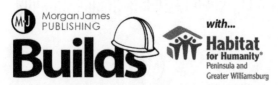

In an effort to support local communities, raise awareness and funds, Morgan James Publishing donates a percentage of all book sales for the life of each book to Habitat for Humanity Peninsula and Greater Williamsburg.

Get involved today! Visit
www.MorganJamesBuilds.com

Dedication

D
r. Joe Hufanda dedicates this book to his parents, Vince and Necitas Hufanda, for instilling in him a higher sense of purpose; to his loving wife, Tanja, who has been supportive of all his undertakings; to Dr. Gary Imm, Dr. Allan Ringard, and Brandon Allen for their friendship, mentoring, and tough love; and to his business partner, Dr. Christian Yaste, who has been the driving force on their many dental adventures.

Dr. Christian Yaste dedicates this book to his parents, Tom and Michelle Yaste, for their unconditional love and encouragement during his journey; to Pastors Minner Labrador, John Bradshaw, and Bryan Aalborg for awakening in him a higher purpose; to Dr. Tony Feck and Dr. Matt Vandermolen for their sound advice and faith in their vision; to his wife, Gabriela, for standing by his side, for always loving, and always believing; and to Dr. Joe Hufanda, whose conscientious foresight made this book possible.

Table of Contents

Chapter 1

Just How Important Are Your Teeth Anyway?

Fix your mouth, change your life!

The joke goes, "An artist and a scientist walk into a bar…."
As for us—Yaste and Hufanda—one of us is a talented
artist and the other has a propensity for science and
engineering. And bars? Well, we haven't had a lot of time for
them.

Dental school was tough and demanding. We each
encountered significant challenges along our journey, bringing
us now to more than two decades of contributing to the dental

health and well-being of thousands we have been privileged to serve. Through the ongoing pursuit of excellence, we have created a dental practice that we'd want for ourselves, our families, and our friends—a dental practice that puts patients front and center.

Your smile and oral health are about how your teeth look, about how everything in your mouth fits together, whether it's a crown, a bridge, a denture, dental implants, veneers, or fillings. Your mouth influences the way you feel about yourself. Your mouth affects your self-image. So the idea of art-meets-construction isn't so far-fetched, is it? It takes both artistry and engineering to create an ideal smile and a healthy mouth. Over the past twenty years we have seen time and time again that people with a healthy smile and mouth have a better quality of life.

The story of a patient who washed cars for a living at a Chevrolet dealership is one of the most significant we can tell you in terms of life-changing events. Brian was a bright young man who washed cars day in and day out. He came to us because he was ashamed of his smile. As a young man he had not taken very good care of his teeth. He had serious problems and cavities everywhere—but it wasn't entirely his fault.

What many people don't realize is the role that genetics plays in our teeth. Of course, neglect can contribute to unhealthy outcomes. You know the saying, "You don't have to floss all your teeth, just the ones you want to keep." Even so, we know personal practice is not the whole picture. Brian's issues were a combination of genetics and neglect.

He came to us in desperation. "I just can't live with it anymore!" he exclaimed. We knew we had to do our best to help him. **In reality, the poor condition of his teeth and mouth had actually changed the course of his life.**

Because he was so self-conscious about his teeth, he would turn his head away or cover his mouth when speaking. Customers at the car dealership viewed him as not interested or less than trustworthy. Brian's bosses saw him the same way, so he was really stuck in a job that was far beneath his potential— and far short of his dreams. His coworkers interpreted his body language and behavior as antisocial and aloof, which was underscored by the fact that he'd never join them for lunch or a beer after work. He was just too embarrassed and worried to relax with them in that way. Can you imagine curtailing your life because you are afraid to smile, speak, and eat around people?

We came up with a comprehensive plan for Brian. However, because he was not making a lot of money, it took some doing to work out all the financial arrangements. Although it was a sacrifice for Brian, he was hopeful it would be worth it. We knew it would be worth it, and we got to work. **How much is your self-image and career worth to you?**

Six or so months passed after the final procedure before we saw Brian again. One day he just showed up at the office to schedule a routine cleaning and check-up. But he had other news he wanted to deliver in person. He told us that after we had renovated his mouth, he couldn't stop smiling at work. His boss soon noticed his endlessly sunny disposition and immediately promoted him to a sales position. Here he would have constant interaction with customers. Apparently, he did so well selling cars that he was promoted again! This time, it was to the finance department, which his boss said was more of a challenge, but one he knew Brian could handle. Excelling there, Brian eventually became finance manager, quadrupling his former car-washing salary.

As if that part of the fairy tale wasn't enough, later he married a beautiful young woman and now has three children. The icing on the cake is that he ended up doing some radio spots for our practice on the merits of good dental care, telling the world (or at least the listening audience) his story! His whole life changed because of one thing: his smile.

A different client of ours was seventy years old when he made an appointment, admitting he hadn't brushed his teeth for half a century! The last time he had seen the dentist was when he was released from the Army after the Korean War. When we looked in his mouth, there was plaque and tartar everywhere. In fact, you couldn't really tell what were teeth and what was tartar. The plaque had turned rock hard! Although we were not worried about being able to help him, this kind of neglect has the potential to cause serious oral and other health problems for many people (see Chapter 4). But when we cleaned him up, we found he had no cavities and no gum disease! What other explanation is there for this than good genes?

In our dental practice we occasionally see the "poster child" patients (or poster *adult*, as our practice focuses on adults) who model diligent self-care, religiously brushing and flossing multiple times a day, and coming in for regular cleanings and check-ups. But regardless of their good habits, they still experience considerable tooth issues and gum disease. While good oral health practices are important, sometimes the hand we're dealt in the first place complicates things. If you have relatives with "bad" teeth, there is a chance you could have the same problems, no matter how diligently you care for your smile.

While not everyone's story is quite as dramatic as Brian's, many come close. And even if your story isn't life-changing, think about how much your teeth mean to you on a daily basis. We have patients who come to us having avoided certain foods—and pleasant experiences—for years. They are unable to enjoy an ice cream cone with their child or grandchild because of pain and sensitivity. Or they shy away from healthy nuts, fresh fruit, and raw vegetables, and some of life's great culinary pleasures, such as a crusty baguette or hearty pizza crust— because they cannot chew without pain.

When it comes to your teeth, we find most of you want three things:

1. A nice-looking smile that doesn't embarrass you;
2. The ability to eat the foods you like;
3. A day-to-day life free of pain.

Teeth are often taken for granted until something goes wrong, and that something can impact everything. Your mouth is among your most important assets. Your smile is what makes you inviting and gives you the confidence that makes you more "comfortable in your own skin," as the saying goes. Your smile contributes more than you may be aware of to the quality of your life.

What matters most

In our practice, both of us bring different strengths and passions to the table, and even though our personalities are different, we share important core values and beliefs. Our patients find it interesting that we've been friends most of our lives, meeting in eighth grade, then attending the same high school. We then went through dental school together and eventually founded the Ballantyne Center for Dentistry in Charlotte, North Carolina.

Among the core values we consider first and foremost is the pursuit of greatness. Giving 100 percent is extremely important to what we do, and we encourage the people who work with us, and for us, to do the same. Our second fundamental value is an emphasis on efficiency. Time is the most valuable asset we all have, and we strive not to waste ours or yours. The third is a strong sense of teamwork. We currently have thirty dedicated individuals on our team, and we all mutually encourage one another to live out our values so our patients benefit from a caring, cohesive culture.

We also consider humility and accountability part of the equation for success, with compassion, respect, loyalty, integrity, and empowerment rounding out our core group of values—just as important as any of the others. We want our patients to have the kind of experience that supersedes any fear or reluctance they may have felt about going to the dentist in the first place, which we will address in greater detail in Chapter 2.

If "listening" were considered a core value, it would definitely be at the top of our list. Listening may be the most important thing we do as dentists. It's important to hear our patients' chief concerns and address those first. We collect as much of the diagnostic information as we can when a patient first comes in. This helps us to develop the right program, meet their financial needs, and figure out a suitable time frame for any work they need done.

One of our older patients—we'll call her "Laura"—came in with a litany of issues, all of which added up to an inability to eat all the wonderful foods, including fried chicken, that she'd be tempted to eat at a family reunion in two months. She also found it difficult to laugh and express her joy while hiding her teeth. Who would want to attend a family reunion where you had to hold back your emotions?

We couldn't fix everything in that two-month time period, and to be honest, she didn't want to fix everything. But we did enough corrective and cosmetic work so that she was able to attend the reunion, smile and laugh without reservation, and partake of the fried chicken family recipe that was as much a part of who she was as her smile. Her smile wasn't perfect, but it was good enough to correct her chief concerns and stay within her budget. When she returned, she counted the days between dental appointments to finish the work. Laura was eager to become a shining example of what's possible in 21st-century dentistry—all in time for next year's reunion!

While Laura wanted everything we could possibly do to improve the quality of her life, timing is everything, and we don't believe in pressuring patients into services they don't need or want. We start by treating issues that are the highest priority for them. Though we look at the big picture, our focus is to fit the recommended procedures into people's budgets and lifestyles.

We've lost track of how many patients come through our door saying they've been seeing Doctor So-and-So for the past ten years, and they are not happy. Most of the time the reason they are not happy is that their current dentist doesn't listen to their concerns. Rather, *they have been told* what their priorities should be. We believe there's an art and balance in listening to patients, acknowledging what's important to them, leading them down the appropriate pathway based on our experience, and making options fit their parameters whenever we can.

We believe in providing information. Here is an example:

Sometimes when a tooth-saving procedure is considered too costly, a patient might ask for the tooth to be pulled instead of repaired. Another dentist may offer tooth removal as a solution. But often, explanations and important facts about the outcome are not discussed, and the repercussions of that choice can be devastating. Patients should *not* have teeth removed before looking at the big picture, considering what the options are, and having a plan put in place beforehand. That doesn't mean that removing the tooth is the wrong choice. But too often we see patients who have had teeth removed without a plan or knowledge of consequences, and down the road, it costs them a small fortune to fix what has happened, if it can be fixed at all.

There is a particularly damaging process called Combination Syndrome in which the top jaw collapses because there are no back teeth in the jaws. The patient's mouth physically changes, and the only way to fix it is with a particularly uncomfortable and expensive surgery or mouth rehabilitation. We see this phenomenon occur when patients have had teeth pulled over time without realizing they could be dentally disabled. If people were just informed ahead of time that this was in their future, perhaps they'd consider some alternatives to having their teeth—or even a single tooth—pulled. At least they might not postpone treatment until it is too late.

Education is so important, running a close second to listening. We form a partnership with our patients. The patient is the driver or conductor, and we're just making sure patients know where they're going and staying on the tracks, going as fast or slow as they want.

Cost and effect

Dentistry is a service, not a commodity. It's not the same as shopping around for a new appliance, looking for the best price. In dentistry, most of the time you get what you pay for. What you're buying is the dentist's time, ability, and skill level. Most dentists base their fees on what other dentists in the area charge and/or on insurance company reimbursements. While it's important to make sure you're not being gouged, you generally won't find huge disparities in costs among most dentists. It's important not to choose a dentist solely on fees and insurance reimbursement, because while not always the case, the quality of care can be lacking in practices where fees are low, and the work may not be guaranteed.

We encourage prospective patients who are "on the fence" to talk to other patients who have gone through similar procedures. If you go for an initial consultation for dental implants or veneers and say, "But I'm just not sure," a good dentist will offer to put you in touch with another patient who has had the same procedure. Because experience is the best teacher, when you talk with someone who has been there and done that, you hear everything, not just our side of the story. Once that's achieved, it's important to go with your gut. We encourage that because again, above all, dentistry is a service; an experience. It is something you choose and should get the best of. If the trust level between you and your dentist is not high, what happens in the chair may not meet your expectations, no matter what kind of job we do.

For 20 years we have been practicing our craft, bringing together our backgrounds in cosmetic dentistry, sedation dentistry, dental implants, reconstruction, and much more to serve our patients. Over these past twenty years, **we have seen a massive shift in the way dentistry is delivered and how that affects the quality of care you receive.** But no one is talking about it. Some, dare I say most dentists, may not even know that it is happening. But we want you to know. We want you to know before it is too late. Dentistry has changed dramatically and you have in your hands a guidebook to many of those changes.

In this book, through the benefit of our experience, we will provide the foundation for you to access the highest levels of adult dental care. We want you to know:

- exactly what questions to ask your dentist
- how to confront dental fears and phobias and the options available
- when to have customized care to meet your needs and circumstances
- what new technologies and techniques are available

- why your smile is SO important
- how changes in corporate dentistry will affect the type of care you may get
- new discoveries about the mouth/body connection
- that the dental problems you have are probably not your fault!
- how dental implants can safely and affordably renew or replace your smile
- the difference between family dentistry and dentistry *specifically designed* to meet the needs of today's adults and understand the kind of impact various dental procedures can have on your life.

Chapter 2

Don't Go To The Dentist?
You're Not Alone

Just because it doesn't hurt …!

My fear of dentists began when I was in dental school. It was in Michigan, 1992, and I was excited to be there. My current dental partner, Dr. Joe Hufanda, and I were headed to class. I was riding my bicycle and encountered some black ice that sent me catapulting over the handle bars.

The result was a row of cracked and smashed front teeth. I spent my entire day going from clinic to clinic at the dental school, sent here and sent there, essentially feeling tortured by some of the experts who were teaching me my craft: my professors. When it was all over, I was so distraught that dentistry could be so cold and agonizing—and ashamed of how hideous I looked—that I was ready to quit dental school. It was a painful experience on every level—and nobody seemed to care about trying to make me look or feel better!

Since that time, and despite our thriving practice, I've been gun-shy about getting my own dental care. I get sweaty palms ten times over. But because of all that, I have a personal connection with people who have dental fears and phobias, as I am one of them. I know they get sick to their stomach and ride the elevator up and down a number of times before mustering up the courage to walk into the reception area. Not only are they not alone, but I joined their ranks more than twenty years ago. While I wish I'd never had that experience, it gave me a gift: I feel empathy with patients that a lot of dentists will never have.

Painful numbers

Polls find that a little less than half of the American population doesn't go to the dentist at all.[1] Fears run the

---

[1]   Lecia Bushak. "Oral Health Isn't Much of Americans' Concern, Poll Finds," Medicaldaily.com. April 29, 2014. http://www.medicaldaily.com/oral-health-isnt-much-americans-concern-poll-finds-one-third-didnt-see-dentist-last-year-279468

gamut from the thought of pain to the sound of drills and other instruments, to objections to the smells of products used in treatment, to potential costs. With that, and in an effort to overcome the blocks, a strong element of trust is integral to any patient-dentist relationship. Even if you visit a practice without dental fear, anxiety, or phobia, any doubt or a lack of faith in what the dentist recommends or how the dentist and staff handle your concerns can cause you to have an experience far beneath what it should be. In fact, a negative experience can cultivate a fear that didn't exist before, as it did with the fallout from my bike accident.

Interestingly, one of the primary reasons people don't go to the dentist routinely is a *lack* of pain. Most often, when a visit looms ahead, it's because the teeth are creating a level of pain you can't turn off and with which you just cannot function anymore. So you call—begging to be squeezed in for an appointment—just to be put out of your misery! But in the early stages of cavities, gum disease, or other potentially painful and detrimental oral conditions, you may not have pain or discomfort. The only action that can determine what is present in your mouth—and what stage it's in—is preventive care. That means regular dental visits and scheduled cleanings, where an exam is performed and x-rays may be taken (depending on when they were last taken). For most people, though, a common mantra is, "If it ain't broke, don't fix it."

To make matters worse, as humans, many of us are creatures of habit. Even a dental emergency doesn't always make us reevaluate the way we manage our teeth. Over and over, we see patients get to a stable point following a dental emergency, but then the pattern continues. "If nothing hurts right now, why go back?"

* * *

A lot of people ask how long it takes for a "tooth event" to evolve—to begin to cause pain. Unfortunately, the answer is as varied as the problems. Everyone is different, and there are different physical forces at work on everyone's teeth. There are genetic links. There are oral flora—meaning the good and bad balance of bacteria and mouth acid—that comes into play. If two people are standing side-by-side, each having a small cavity lesion, one could progress fairly quickly and in a year require a root canal. The other could take years to reach that point. There are many determinants to how the cavity develops, and everyone's are different.

The fact is, dentistry used to be a real pain-driven business. Sixty or so years ago, you really didn't go to the dentist unless you had pain. Dentists were always more or less "putting out fires." After World War II, the enterprising Bristol-Myers

Company developed a concept that people should go to the dentist every six months for a check-up and cleaning. Remember the company's Ipana toothpaste campaign—"Brusha, brusha, brusha"—and its pitchman, Bucky Beaver? Over the years, we discovered just how gum disease works and why people lose their teeth—all the reasons we've talked about, including bacterial infections, acid erosion, force, and genetics. There are some cases where trauma comes in, such as a bike or car accident, or other instances where teeth can be damaged. But in general, preventative care is the way to maintain good oral health, just as having an annual physical and other diagnostics, including prostate exams and mammograms, is the best way to head off the potential for illness and disease.

Drill and fill

As Baby Boomers came on the scene, common practice was to fill the patient's mouth with metal if they had a cavity. Alloy fillings containing mercury—called "amalgams"—were used. The rule for design was called "extension for prevention": dentists would drill out the tooth decay and put in a metal filling. The idea was that the more we undercut and extended the size of the preparation, the better the filling would stay in the tooth.

Unfortunately, we have learned that, over several decades, amalgam fillings expand and contract, causing fractures in the teeth and allowing bacteria to leak in underneath, creating more tooth decay. These teeth will crack, which can be painful and costly to fix. Many times, if someone waits until the tooth begins to develop symptoms, they learn it will need a root canal, build-ups, or possibly even extraction! Preventative therapy can be so much less painful and so much more cost-effective.

Recently we saw a woman in our practice who was one of the "victims" of this early thinking in dentistry. She wasn't so keen on dentists because of the negative experiences she'd had in her childhood. Her mouth was clearly the product of mediocre dentistry. When she came to us, she was also predisposed to acid and bacterial infections. There were neglect issues, and frankly, she had used narcotics to an extreme, which had dried out her mouth, making it more susceptible to tooth decay. All her old metal fillings were falling apart. We had to remove all her teeth and use dental implants to restore her mouth back to health. It was a very costly process, but through it, her faith in dentistry was renewed. She has vowed to keep up with her dental care from this point on.

Periodontal (gum) disease: the silent killer

In literature, someone referred to as "long in the tooth" is typically a wise and respected elder. But the fact is that long-looking teeth are generally caused by receding gums and/or gum disease. There are some people who even have this condition as young adults, though it is most commonly diagnosed as a condition of aging. Some statistics show that as many as 60 percent of individuals over forty years old who see a dentist regularly have mild to advanced forms of gum disease. Periodontal surgeries also can make the gums shrink back. In time, the foundation of the bone is lost and teeth start shifting—especially if one or two teeth have to be extracted. In fact, your sinus can drop down, creating a wide range of additional problems. Over time, your face can actually collapse. Yet some people who are fearful or reticent about going to the dentist when all this is happening prefer to throw caution to the wind and "let nature take its course"—or any of a hundred other clichés that mean avoidance and subsequent disaster.

Years ago, we had a patient who ultimately faced this situation head-on. Although we explained that he could probably get a couple more years out of his teeth if he came in for more frequent cleanings and maintained them well on his own, he elected to hedge his bets and opt instead for dental implants. Often, this is actually the least risky and most cost-effective way to restore a mouth to health and avoid other medical problems that can be caused or exacerbated by gum disease (which we talk about in Chapter 4). We ended up using dental implants in the upper and the lower jaws with a beautiful porcelain prosthesis that looked and functioned better than our patient's natural teeth had. For him, having this work done was the best investment he could make. He no longer suffered from pain and discomfort, and he was able to enjoy a beautiful smile designed just for him.

As an international salesman who traveled extensively, he needed assurance that he wasn't going to be embarrassed by a tooth breaking down and flying out of his mouth, or inconvenienced by tooth pain in some remote area of the globe. He's now enjoying all the confidence that comes with a healthy mouth and amazing smile.

The root of it

Sometimes people experience dental anxiety that is not about pain, but instead about money. Our international salesman patient used to joke that, when all was said and done, he'd put the equivalent of a BMW into his mouth. But we can tell you from experience that if a patient doesn't address a burgeoning problem, the cost will be far greater than it is at the outset or even in the middle of a serious dental problem.

We follow patients who were diagnosed in the dental hygiene department with periodontal disease. They may say it's just not in the budget at that point to do anything about it. They've got kids in college or they just bought a house. But over the next three to five years, we're talking about doing a denture. Once again, they believe there is no pain, so why go to the expense of taking any measures, right? In time, there's major bone loss, and sometimes it's too late to keep the teeth because there's no longer a secure foundation, due to the destruction caused by periodontal disease. They are forced to decide on other options—fewer and perhaps less preferable than if they'd taken steps when the problem was first diagnosed.

But wait–there is hope!

With today's technology, patients may not have to settle for something they absolutely don't want, just because of economics. Twenty years ago, some patients had to settle for dentures when they were a less expensive treatment option. Some patients ended up stuck with them, no matter how depressing it was. Today, even people with limited budgets can afford dental implants, which are considered a much better option. It may have to be done over time—and yes, they may have to reprioritize and not take their grandchildren to Disney World for a couple more years or put off remodeling the kitchen, or they may have to maintain an older car a little longer. But there are options, and good ones. We are now able to work out a lot of financing through our creative treatment planning—something that dentists didn't typically do a couple of decades ago—to make excellent dental care more attainable. You might say that in that respect, we are completely fearless!

Smorgasbord of smile options

We like to think we have a "black belt" in multi-disciplinary care. In the past, many general dentists who would see someone with moderate periodontal disease would recommend pulling the tooth or teeth that were involved and giving the patient a denture or partial denture. There was no other way. But now, because of the advanced technology and training available to dentists treating adult patients, we can provide better solutions. We might suggest a "dental collage" (and here's where our art and building backgrounds referenced in Chapter 1 kick in). These are elements that come together to make for an aesthetically pleasing mouth. It also makes for a happy heart when you look in the mirror! A preemptive strike may be worth its weight in gold … er … or titanium, if you opt for dental implants!

It's really a big-picture thing. Many dentists treat teeth, so that's what they focus on, instead of zooming out and looking more comprehensively or holistically. They fail to go for the panoramic view. (Think *BIG* picture here.) But as dentists focused on treating adult patients, we try to look at the whole person—at the causes of pain, deterioration, and discomfort that are not always obvious.

Let's draw a parallel. If you have a house and are looking to fix things and also remodel, what would happen if you just replaced pipes and put on an addition without examining the foundation? Before doing new work, you have to back up considerably and look at the whole project. Laserlike focus and attention to detail are great, but not without a 360-degree view.

We have patients who have come to us over the years from other general family practices where their former dentist kept filling cavity after cavity after cavity. There was something going on, but the dentist never seemed to take the time to ferret it out. Or perhaps their teeth kept breaking and requiring an awful lot of repair. Those dentists were like home remodelers buying a new pipe without figuring out the underlying problem. They just kept fixing and replacing without venturing deeper into the patient's situation. What was causing the deterioration of the teeth to begin with?

With one patient in particular, we wondered why the previous dentist had not ever questioned her bite. Once we fixed it, she never broke another tooth. Though it may sound incongruous, a big part of effective dentistry is similar to being a detective or an investigative journalist. This level of care can help patients overcome their fears and phobias and restore confidence about going to the dentist. To be fair, many family dentists are so busy treating teeth for so many patients in so many age groups that they use a less effective model of care in their practice. They might not realize their adult patients need more TLC. We will discuss this in greater detail very soon.

Judge not lest ye be judged

Another side of "dental resistance," to coin a term, is fear of intimidation or judgment. In more than two decades in practice, we've come across our share of dental practices that operate by essentially *instilling* fear and humiliation. Some dentists imply that if a patient doesn't conform to their way of doing things (with few or no options presented), and incur the expense involved, the world will come to an end—or the patient's world will. In our opinion, there is no room for tactics like this in dentistry. But there should be a balance involved, a formula that includes what a patient really needs and expects and what can be done for them within their comfort zone—in terms of both experience and dollars.

If a patient comes to us with markedly ugly teeth, but that individual is comfortable with them, we are not going to impose an absolute course of action on him. We may recommend a treatment plan but also say, "If you feel good about yourself and are happy with the way things are, and there is no element of disease that needs attention, so be it." Conversely, someone with really beautiful teeth can come in and express dismay about an almost imperceptible chip, insisting it be fixed, and we'll take care of it. Everybody's different. No two people's expectations or philosophies are exactly the same.

Some dentists are afraid to address deeper issues with a patient because they think it compromises the patient's personal space, or it might be an uncomfortable discussion. If a patient reacts curiously to a suggestion, it might be perfectly normal for them, or it may be a manifestation of some kind of fear or phobia. In many cases, it behooves the dentist to probe a little to get to know their patient better, ensuring the best possible course of treatment, experience, and long-term outcome. We often say, if all you have in your tool belt is a hammer, everything looks like a nail. It's better for a dentist to take the extra step of knowing exactly who their patient is. That way, if they cannot provide the appropriate solution, they can at least be a trusted advisor and help patients find a solution somewhere else.

A friend and colleague of ours coined the term "dental disabilities" some years ago to refer to a situation in which some dental condition affects the way you see yourself. Your mouth can affect your self-confidence—your ability to function in the world as a whole person. Some people are depressed because they don't like how their mouth looks, so they will not go out with their friends or even family, in some cases. Others deal with the discomfort of their replacement teeth but wonder whether, if they join their friends for lunch, they will be able to eat what's on the menu. Some may not be confident of their dental adhesive's longevity, so they don't go out for fear of their dentures coming loose and slipping at an inopportune time. Given all these hassles and inconveniences, going out in public can be torture for people with dental problems.

Earlier in the book, we talked about Brian, the car-washer-turned-finance-department-manager whose personal relationships and professional life changed in every respect when his teeth did. A spectacular dental office culture will reflect more nurturing and listening than other practices may. These dental practices tend to have more than just hammers in their professional tool belts, so fewer things look like a nail. Not every dentist is the same—or as we like to say, a dentist is not a dentist is not a dentist. Finding one with the skill set and mindset to help with the specific problems you may have—including your fears and anxieties—is imperative for a great outcome.

We are not the only dentists who think this way. There are dentists in almost every community who have a similar mindset. Your objective should be to take the time to find one, because a dentist's philosophy is not always dependent on age, experience, or how glamorous the office is. Later on in the book, we will explore how to find the right dentist for your particular circumstances.

Chapter 3

How the Interaction Between the General Practitioner and Specialist Has Changed Today

What it means for you

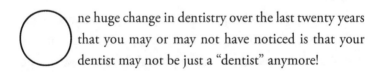ne huge change in dentistry over the last twenty years that you may or may not have noticed is that your dentist may not be just a "dentist" anymore!

The way we were

Many of us grew up in a time when dentistry was separated into a range of specialties and specialists. There was, of course, the general family dentist. That was the dentist to whom you went for check-ups, fillings, and other basic dental care. If you needed braces, your dentist referred you to the orthodontist. If you needed your wisdom teeth pulled, you were sent to an oral surgeon. For a root canal, you were set up with an appointment for an endodontist. Gum disease meant a trip to a periodontist. Later on, as specialties evolved, if you wanted your mouth rebuilt, you might have been referred to a prosthodontist.

It used to be that the top 10 percent of a dental school graduating class was expected to go on to a specialty. These elite students were considered the brightest—the chosen ones—and were more likely to be accepted into specialty dental education because of their high grades. Most of these individuals would spend an additional two to four years learning a particular specialty.

But that's all changing now. Specialty programs, while still present, are becoming less and less appealing to graduating dental students because so many general dentists now can do it all. In addition, the average dental student graduates with an average of over $260,000 worth of student loan debt right out of the starting gate, and they don't want to go to school for another two to three years, incurring more debt. Dentists in the 21st century are just not as interested in pursuing the specialty path as dentists once were. Most now opt for *a la carte* training instead, in what used to be considered areas of specialty.

The general dentist becomes the 'Super GP'

Among the factors that have made it feasible for general dentists today to do it all—or at least a lot of it—are great strides in readily available technology. This includes diagnostic aids, lasers, microscopes, cad-cam units, scanners, digital radiography, and so much more. Additionally, there is advanced postgraduate training through continuing education available for general dentists to learn specific specialty procedures. Dental consultants have begun to call dentists reaching out into this new territory "Super General Practitioners." These advancements have changed the landscape of dentistry significantly. In this chapter, we will explain what this big change means for you.

Seeing a general dentist who is trained in multiple specialty procedures can offer real advantages for an adult patient— convenience, continuity, and accountability being the most obvious. But in some instances, including a dental specialist in a patient's care is still the best choice. To clarify how general dentists and dental specialists work both together and separately, let's look at the example of a dental implant procedure.

There's a wide range of options and protocols in the implants arena, and a wealth of knowledge is necessary. Implants involve a complex, multifaceted process. In the past—in fact, only a few short years ago—it was almost always necessary for a general dentist and a specialist to work together to provide this type of complex dentistry.

The general dentist would send a patient they thought might be a candidate for a dental implant to the oral surgeon (specialist). The surgeon would then complete the surgical phase of treatment and refer the patient back to their general dentist, who would finish the procedure. It was crucial for communication between the general dentist, who was doing the restorative work—and the specialist, who began by extracting the tooth or teeth, and placing the bone graft and dental implant—to go smoothly. Otherwise, there was the potential for not only a negative patient experience, but a less-than-desired clinical result.

The main reason for engaging with a specialist was that typically, general dentists did not completely understand the surgical side of the process and had never been taught how to do it. Today, in light of the changes mentioned earlier—specifically those in technology and the postgraduate courses available to general dentists—it is becoming more and more common that your dentist is acutely aware of your dental implant options. And in many practices, dentists are actually performing the entire dental implant procedure under one roof, without the need to refer a patient to a specialist.

But something still holds true today, as it has in the past: in order to achieve a successful result when a general dentist refers a patient to a dental specialist, there needs to be one captain— one "general contractor," so to speak. Typically it would be the general dentist who is in charge, assuming the responsibility for the final product. When the general dentist doesn't take charge, patients tend to feel abandoned and confused, wondering what is next and who is supposed to be doing what. This is a common frustration and generally leaves a bad taste in patients' mouths—no pun intended.

As mentioned, dental implants are a complex and multifaceted procedure, so even the general dentist who focuses on just the restorative phase should have a deep understanding of how the surgical process works. This is intrinsic to an optimal outcome.

We have learned (and usually perform) both phases of the dental implant procedure: the surgical and the restorative. We obtained this advantage through particularized coursework, postgraduate courses, and other forms of continuing education, as well as investments in technology.

Although the proliferation of accessible education and increasingly affordable technology has provided a real boost for dentists to be able to provide specialty care for their patients, much of the push for general dentists to do the entire procedure by themselves was sparked by the arrival of middle-aged Baby Boomers. This discerning group did not want to be without teeth, and they wanted one place to have their dental needs met. The "one-stop-shopping" mindset has become increasingly popular during the past few years, especially with adults who have more complex dental needs.

Here is a fact you may find interesting. A few decades ago, dental specialists didn't know how to put in dental implants because they hadn't been taught the procedure as part of their post-dental-school specialty training. Unless they took specific postgraduate courses, they'd never have learned how to do it. But today, general dentists have access to the same postgrad courses as specialists did, so it's not as if the general practitioner can't obtain the same breadth and scope of knowledge.

So how and when do patients know they might need a specialist versus a general dentist? For one thing, we've always advocated the patient asking a lot of questions.

Again, let's use dental implants as an example, though any specialty treatment can be substituted. You might ask these questions:

- How much of this procedure do you do? (Ask for specific numbers, i.e., "How many dental implants do you place every year?")
- What is the brand of the implant you would be using, and why did you choose it?
- Is this a regular part of your practice?
- How many years have you been doing it? How long has this implant system and the company that makes it been on the market? (If an implant company goes out of business, sometimes parts cannot be obtained down the road if a maintenance procedure becomes necessary.)
- Can I talk with some of your patients who have had this procedure done?
- What about your staff? Do you do their dental work, and have you performed this procedure on any of them? Is there someone in the office with whom I can have a conversation?

So much of the decision to have a procedure done in-house or to seek out a specialist depends on the diagnostician—or the dentist. Your general dentist should know his or her limitations and what procedures would get the same results, whether performed by a specialist or by themselves. A trustworthy dentist will let you know how comfortable he is with the procedure and whether it is within his skill set. If it is a procedure with which she is less than comfortable, the dentist should refer you to a specialist to whom she would send her own friends and family members. This is very important. Just ask.

The shiny new dentist

If you're seen by dentists straight out of dental school, you hope they've paid attention, gotten high marks, and learned a lot. But sometimes experience goes a lot farther than the education part. In fact, most of the dental skills we wield today were skills we acquired *after* graduating from dental school! That being said, sometimes even experience and education are no match for common sense and the ability to implement what has been learned.

So if your dentist is just out of school or even a couple of years into the practice, the odds are that he or she may refer you to a specialist for some non-routine procedures—but not always. There are some young dentists who are highly motivated and incredibly talented. When a dentist like this has the appropriate mentorship, coaching, and training, they can often become "Super GPs" in far less time than their colleagues who have had years of experience.

Greater convenience, better communication

A significant benefit of having a complex procedure handled by one capable and highly skilled practitioner is the accountability factor. We've seen situations where two or even three dentists involved in a single case, who might be very good practitioners, failed to achieve a patient's desired result due to a lack of communication or a miscommunication among them. A great advantage to having a procedure executed by the same dentist is that the proverbial buck stops there.

In a practice like ours, with four decades of experience and countless hours of continuing education between us, we try to keep procedures in-office. This allows us to make things more convenient for patients and also have more control over the results. We have found most individuals are looking for one place to have most, if not all, of their procedures done.

Certifiable?

People sometimes ask about certifications. They are important. If dentists are board-certified, it certainly indicates they've invested the time in education and gone the distance with the testing involved.

The next fact may be somewhat confusing, but it is important to note. While general dentists can be certified and licensed as such by their respective state licensing boards, they cannot be claim to specialize in any particular dental specialty—even if they routinely include endodontic or periodontal work or some oral surgery in their practices. They can, on the other hand, receive certification in continuing education courses for specialties, as we have done. (As an interesting aside, currently no board certification exists for several types of specialty procedures, including dental implants and cosmetic dentistry.)

That dentist has quite the reputation!

One of the most important determinants of where to have a procedure done and who should be doing it are the questions we talked about earlier, but let's not forget the dentist's reputation. A reputation can take years to build and moments to destroy. Today it is easy to assess a dentist's reputation. The Internet has made it easy to find out what people think of your dentist—or anyone else's, for that matter. Google, Yelp, Healthgrades.com, and other websites are excellent resources to discover just what people are saying. The best dentists are acutely aware of this and will strive to make not only a good first impression, but also to provide top-notch care every time you visit.

In our office, we ask patients for two things. First, if we do something wrong, or in any way make you uncomfortable, please let us know personally. Everyone on our team is empowered to take care of a patient who has a question, complaint, or problem.

And second, if we do something right, please let everyone else know! Tell your friends and family members that you had a stellar experience with us so that they know our office is a safe and comfortable place to have their dentistry done. Fourteenth and fifteenth century monk and poet John Lydgate said, "You can please some of the people all of the time, you can please all of the people some of the time, but you can't please all of the people all of the time." In the 21st century, Drs. Yaste and Hufanda say, "The best dentists aim to please all of the people as many times as possible!"

Danger: the newbie expert

There are some instances where a general dentist will attend a weekend seminar and become an "expert" within that short period of time. Have you seen the commercial that was popular a few years ago about the kind of authority, expert, or super-achiever that staying at a Holiday Inn Express the night before makes you? If you haven't, type that into Google for a hearty laugh.

Unfortunately, we have seen this phenomenon become more prevalent during the past few years. A few dentists are in a rush to keep up with the changes in technology and are trying to become that "Super GP" as quickly as they can. The unfortunate thing is that it's hard to know if a dentist is actually an expert unless you start asking the questions we mentioned earlier in the chapter. Would you let an electrician wire your house after two days of study? It might be tempting, in a cost-savings kind of way—but unless you're partial to spur-of-the-moment campfires, it's probably not worth rolling the dice. The same applies when it comes to your teeth. So just be careful that you ask the right questions and research the dentist's reputation.

'Just look at my teeth!'

Earlier, we touched upon inquiring of a staff member at the office who may have had the procedure done that you are considering. Sometimes patients don't think about it, but asking an employee if the dentists in the office treat their own staff members—and more importantly, if members of the staff would even *consider* having their boss(es) work on their mouths—is extremely revealing. It might be a giant red flag as to whether you should have a specialty procedure provided by that dentist.

We have a friend who is a very good dentist. He recently purchased a practice from a retiring dentist. As soon as he took over, every single employee approached him with a sigh of relief, saying they'd finally feel comfortable getting their own dental work done there. They hadn't trusted their former boss's clinical skills. If the team feels that way and will be candid with you, you can make a much more informed decision.

Years ago, an astute, older dentist shared a secret with us. He told us one of the biggest investments we can ever make is to spend the time and money to do dentistry for the individuals who work for us. "If they're happy and trust you, they'll talk about it," he said emphatically. If a patient in the chair is wavering on a procedure and mentions it to the hygienist or another staff person, happy team members will invariably encourage the patient to go ahead with it, because they've had the work done themselves. They can talk the prospective patient through the whole thing, complete with recovery time, any pain management necessary, accolades, and everything else—and it's all first-hand information. This has proven to be an invaluable resource for us. Staff recommendations are especially helpful when we present treatment options that patients might consider more of a specialty procedure.

If a dentist doesn't treat his or her employees, they often have no success stories to tell that readily come to mind, especially at that pivotal moment when it may count for a patient. In advertising, nothing sells weight-loss products like a formerly-overweight-but-currently-svelte spokesperson in a swimsuit who has used the product. In restaurants, food is often sold based on the server's recommendations. So the smart establishments make sure employees try out their goods and services. It's no different in dentistry. In many cases, all the team member has to do is smile widely and say, "Dr. Yaste/ Dr. Hufanda did my smile" to increase the patient's confidence, comfort level, and resulting commitment to the procedure.

So from a patient's perspective, inquiring of the team if their dental work was done in-house—and what those procedures consisted of—can tell you much of what you need to know about whether to keep it local or find a specialist for work that is more complex.

At the end of the day, all dentists—general practitioners and specialists—should be held to a similar standard of care. There are some exceptions, such as in rural areas where dental specialists may not be available, or if a procedure needs to be done quickly and scheduling with a specialist may not be a timely option. Otherwise, the general dentist should place an implant, do a root canal, or perform any other specialty procedure only if he or she is fully qualified and will follow the same protocol as the specialist. If general dentists have acquired the appropriate clinical skills, they can assume full responsibility.

In our practice, we believe if we're going to do something, we're going to have all the diagnostic aids, tools, and experience to make it work. Otherwise, we will help our patients find a practitioner who can provide the most appropriate care.

Chapter 4

Great Health Starts With Great Dental Health

The mouth-body connection—is it real?

In addition to the joy and self-confidence of being able to flash a beautiful smile, being healthy overall can be directly related to what was going on inside your mouth. Though it may be a novel concept for some, in many cases, great health really does start with great dental health!

One risk factor for poor resulting health is a dry mouth. This is also known as xerostomia: a low volume of saliva present in the mouth. Low saliva flow may result in loss of protection of your teeth and gums. If you do not have enough saliva, bacteria will grow in larger amounts, which can make you more susceptible to gum disease and tooth decay that impact your body. Saliva also buffers the pH levels of the mouth and prevents acid erosion of the teeth, so you need to be producing enough of it.

There are several culprits that cause dry mouth. Certain types of medications, alongside radiation and chemotherapy treatments for cancer, can cause dry mouth. Combinations of other commonly taken medications have also been known to contribute to low production of saliva. Autoimmune diseases such as Sjogren's syndrome can cause the condition as well.

Most people understand that bacteria in the mouth can lead to cavities and gum disease, but high acid levels can also be a big problem. Some foods, including those high in acid, can erode tooth enamel, affecting oral health and, by association, overall health. One thing we like our patients to know is the importance of reducing acidity in their mouths as well as in their bodies. Just as higher acid levels in the body, which can be caused by inflammation and the food and drink we consume, can increase the propensity for disease, higher levels of acid in the mouth can create significant dental problems.

A source of acid that some may not be aware of are the electrolyte replacement drinks that are so popular with some people who are active in sports. And it seems today we're constantly snacking or subscribing to the concept of "six small meals a day" to maintain blood glucose levels. But if you never stop eating long enough to let your saliva buffer the acid that's being produced from the kinds of food you've put in your mouth, it will never produce the neutralizing solution that circulates and recalcifies the teeth.

Acid is particularly dangerous around dental work because there is a very small gap between dental work and your natural tooth. Acid attacks the interface between your dental work and the tooth, which allows bacteria to get in and makes the restoration break down faster than it should. Just as the body is better off in a more balanced and buffered state, so is the mouth.

In the beginning

When things aren't working well in the mouth, it can be a gateway to compromised health in other areas of the body. There are several different categories of disease and systemic health problems that may have their beginnings in dental disease, although it is important to note the conversation changes frequently about where disease originates. And though disease can start with conditions in the mouth and impact the body, sometimes it works in reverse: poor oral health may be caused by something going on in the body first, such as a weakened immune system. Low immune function can cause oral fungal and viral infections. Diabetes may contribute to bleeding gums, dry mouth, fungal infections, and cavities, even if patients are diligent about caring for their teeth.

Risk factors for heart disease—to use a strong example—are sometimes linked to one's state of oral health. In 2009, The Academy of General Dentistry published an article on the link between periodontal disease and cardiovascular disease. Forms of cardiovascular disease—a condition reported to affect more than 80 million people a year in the United States—include high blood pressure, acute heart attack, angina pectoris, stroke, and heart failure. As chronic inflammation and infections of the gums and surrounding tissue are indicators of periodontal disease, some research tells us bacteria associated with oral health problems can enter the bloodstream and impact the cardiovascular system.[2]

It has also been suggested that inflammation from periodontal disease can play a role in the formation of blood clots. Clots decrease blood flow to the heart, and when clots become dislodged from the source, they can end up in the lungs (as pulmonary emboli). If it travels to the brain, a clot

[2]   Bhairavi P. Sheth, DMD.

can cause a stroke.3 Again, it can be hard to tell "what comes first, the chicken or the egg?" when discussing cardiovascular disease causing dental health issues, or vice versa. Maintaining a healthy mouth is an important part of optimal health, leaving much less to chance. As one expert put it, "The few minutes you spend a day brushing and flossing is a small price to pay to not have bypass surgery when you are older if there does turn out to be a connection."4

According to 2013 Mayo Clinic-published findings, poor oral health—specifically periodontitis—in pregnant women has been cited as a cause for premature birth and low birth weight. Osteoporosis may be linked to periodontal bone and tooth loss. Finally, endocarditis—a rare infection of the heart's inner lining, or endocardium—can occur when bacteria from other parts of the body, including the mouth, spread through the bloodstream and attach to damaged areas of the heart.5

---

3   3 "The link between gum health and heart disease," last modified June 2016, Delta Dental. https://www.deltadentalins.com/oral_health/heart.html

4   "Mouth and Body Connection," CariFree. http://carifree.com/patient/cavities-a-z/mouth-body-connection.html

5   "What conditions may be linked to oral health?" Last modified March 2016, Mayo Clinic. http://www.mayoclinic.org/healthy-lifestyle/adult-health/in-depth/dental/art-20047475?pg=2

Your teeth and your grandparents' teeth

In presenting all sides of the issue, for some patients genetics plays a role in good (or, on the other side, poor) dental health. While the good genes banner should never be waved as a substitute for prudent routine oral health habits, there are the fortunate few who have come through our office almost like Teflon. No matter what they've done to themselves (or not done), nothing bad sticks—or even occurs in the first place.

As we mentioned in Chapter 1, several years ago we first saw a seventy-year-old man who'd informed us he'd not been to a dentist since he got out of the military—half-a-century earlier! When he opened his mouth, it was impossible to distinguish what was a tooth from what wasn't. There was junk everywhere in the form of caked-on plaque and so much more. We thought for sure we were going to end up taking out all of his teeth and replacing them with dentures, which was what he'd thought, too. But once we chipped all the tartar off his teeth, there wasn't a single cavity or a shred of evidence of gum disease.

So how do you compare him with another patient who brushes and flosses two or three times a day, has regular dental check-ups for years and years, but still has major dental health issues? Apparently our seventy-year-old patient had all the right antibodies and other protective entities in his saliva—so much so that his mouth was impervious to the bad conditions that probably should have developed. We like to say there are some individuals who can brush their teeth with Tootsie Rolls and still emerge with pristine oral health. Unfortunately, most of us are not this lucky.

You are how you feel

When we talk about great dental health having an impact on our overall health, there are psychosocial implications as well. While manifestation of disease in our bodies is one thing, the repercussions of poor dental health can also be found in our state of mind: how we think and how we act. The condition of the mouth can determine where we go (or don't go), what we do (or don't do), and what we achieve or don't achieve in our personal and professional lives. It might even affect the risks we are willing to take to improve ourselves.

Earlier in the book, we talked about Brian, the car-washer-turned-finance- department-manager of a major car dealership whose poor oral health had held him back in life in every way possible. When he addressed the issue, he went through the stratosphere on many levels. We have had many patients who experience the same constraints to varying degrees, the results showing up in lives they choose to limit out of shame and embarrassment. In this regard, even if poor dental health doesn't end up causing cardiovascular or other forms of disease, it can cause self-esteem issues, depression, and other negatives that, over time, become so ingrained in our behavior that our lives are lived in the shadows—or might eventually derail.

But in a world where youth and beauty tend to trump everything else, people are no longer relegated to living with less-than-satisfactory appearances and poor oral health. After a little due diligence, anyone can enlist the help of a good dental practitioner who can partner with him or her to make important changes toward a healthy lifestyle.

Louise

A patient of ours (we'll call her "Louise") had been married for about ten years and, because of the condition of her mouth, hadn't left her house in most of that time. She'd not gone to the grocery store, the movies, out to dinner with her husband— or anywhere. She'd even admitted that it was impossible for her to be physically intimate with him. It was too much of a challenge for her to participate in her children's lives outside the home because of the way she felt about looking the way she did. The way Louise lived, almost like a hermit, was putting a considerable strain on her marriage and family, to say the least. She had severe periodontal disease, missing teeth, a lot of decay, and other manifestations of poor dental health. The woman was barely living—merely existing.

Louise was thoroughly ashamed of her circumstances and said she'd ridden the elevator to our office up and down many times before finally finding the courage to come in. She was unsure we could actually help her. Though she believed her mouth was a complete disaster, we saw an opportunity to change her life. She went through treatment that totally transformed her appearance, her state of mind, and her life. She began wearing make-up again, spruced up her wardrobe, and rejoined society. Today, Louise is living the life she dreamed of. Not only is she a beneficiary of a great transformation in how she looks, thinks, and feels, but her children, husband, and anyone else who interacts with her benefit from it as well. The effects of great dental health can have as much impact on people psychologically as they do physically.

What dental patients want

As we mentioned in Chapter 1, people generally want three things in regard to their oral health:

1. They want to have confidence in their smiles so when the rest of the world looks at them (and judges them, as we all tend to do), they have nothing to hold back—nothing to hide. They can simply shine.
2. They want to be able to eat the foods they love.

3. They want a pain-free mouth.

Taken a step further, whenever possible, you want good dental health that can also help prevent disease elsewhere in your body. Though some may not be aware of the connection at the outset, we do our best to make sure they understand the big picture as we partner with them on the road to great dental health and great health overall.

Chapter 5

Are You Your Own Best 'Dentist' Between Visits?

The self-care you can and should provide

Whether in medicine or dentistry, no one would say it's wise to self-diagnose a problem and act solely on that information. The Internet is so widely used today, it carries a potential danger: patients can plug in a word or a brief description of symptoms—leaving out other information that can, and often does, impact the condition—and receive a diagnosis that may be 180 degrees from the correct one. The Internet can be a real asset, but it can also be a minefield.

You need reliable information from a dental health professional. However, you are still in charge. You are your own best "dentist," only because dentists can't be with patients twenty-four hours a day!

Every treatment should have a *specific* diagnosis first

When it comes to arriving at a diagnosis, our patients generally know what they are experiencing and how they feel. If the dentist doesn't ask all the right questions in carving out a diagnosis, it really is incumbent upon you, the patient, to present the facts as only you can know them. You know your body best. Dentists need to do a significant job of inquiring— and, just as important, *listening*—as you describe what you experience. That is exactly what we do in our practice.

So many factors can inform a diagnosis and the procedure that is needed. Fine distinctions—such as when pain occurs, how long it lasts, the nature of the pain, any sensitivity from heat or cold, the exact location (in dentistry, some pain is referred, and dentists can miss the mark in isolating the right tooth), how intense it is, and what makes it better or worse—can be significant. Being a keen observer of your own oral health gives your dentist important information. Determining the right course of action depends on the quality of interaction that takes place in the dental chair.

The importance of being proactive

It is important for you to take a proactive stance in maintaining your oral health at home. Typically, after a dental cleaning, the hygienist will recommend that you brush at least twice a day and floss once a day (although some research shows biofilm, or slimy bacteria film, can take forty-eight hours to develop, so flossing every other day might be enough). As an alternative to using dental floss, we favor the Hydrofloss™ hydromagnetic oral irrigator, which changes the polarity of your teeth and prevents plaque from sticking to them. Sometimes, as people age, their dexterity diminishes and it becomes more challenging to work with conventional dental floss. Inadequate flossing can hasten decay and gum disease, because biofilm and bacteria are not thoroughly removed. A hydromagnetic oral irrigator provides a real boost in achieving optimal oral health.

Choosing the correct toothpaste or dentifrice can be the key to keeping a healthy mouth. Many of the toothpastes available are merely abrasives, and some toothpaste manufacturers put questionable chemicals and abrasive ingredients in their products primarily for marketing purposes, claiming wondrous results. For the most part, the best toothpaste will be one with lower levels of abrasives. In some cases, it may be best to not even use toothpaste and to instead find a non-alcoholic mouth rinse. We have had patients in our practice who use old-fashioned baking soda to brush their teeth, and guess what? This is actually not a bad idea—if you can get past the taste. The abrasiveness index of straight baking soda is low, so brushing your teeth with plain baking soda is actually quite safe. You may have heard from your dentist that you are brushing your teeth too hard, creating "toothbrush abrasion"—notches in your teeth at the gum line and recession of the gums. But new research shows that this condition is less likely to be caused by how hard you brush and more likely caused by the type of toothpaste you use.

A wide, white, wonderful smile!

If whitening at home is the goal, you should be using a whitening toothpaste featuring an oxygenating or bleaching ingredient—not chemical abrasives that wear away enamel. Whitening is not dangerous to teeth if the agent used acts "from the inside out." Teeth are porous, and a whitening agent will get into those pores, whereas an abrasive will work only on the exterior to remove the stain—plus some of the tooth structure, so it can get at the stain.

Using a hard toothbrush and/or scrubbing excessively hard with any toothbrush is an oral enemy. Some people decide that if they've skipped brushing their teeth a few times, a merciless scrubbing will eradicate everything that's built up. In fact, aggressive scrubbing might do more harm than good. It can abrade tooth enamel and even cause bleeding. We recommend that you always use the softest toothbrush possible.

There are also "designer" toothpastes, mouth rinses, gels, etc.—by that, we mean made with chemical-free or all-natural or herbal products. These might contain an oxygenating ingredient that produces bubbles to power away stains and debris. Most of these are quite good compared to what you may buy at the pharmacy or grocery store (it varies by brand), although designer dental products are typically more expensive. While we are not here to endorse specific products, a little research on your part can reveal a lot.

No need for outlets

Many times, patients ask if electric toothbrushes are better than manual ones. We respond that brushing thoroughly with a manual, soft toothbrush for two minutes, twice a day, achieves the same objective. If you're brushing the right way, that's what matters. Your dental hygienist can tell you what the right way is to brush—angling up toward the gum line or small circles, for example—and also how to floss properly. It can be surprising how many people take their brushing and flossing style for granted, because they've brushed and flossed their whole lives (we hope!). But the hygienist often can show you a more effective way.

Individuals who have lost dexterity in their hands, have arthritis, or need the help of a timer to keep the brush in their mouths for the appropriate two minutes might find an electric brush useful. Often, as we get older, our hands are not as nimble, and having an electric toothbrush do some of the work for you can be quite helpful.

Fear of 'forces'

This is a good fear—the kind you want to have! In addition to brushing and flossing, making sure you're not doing anything in your daily life to damage your teeth is also part of being your own best "dentist." Be aware of what you put into your mouth: chewing on ice, pencils, sticky caramels, gravel-consistency cereals, and other overly crunchy snacks can harm your teeth. Biting off beer bottle caps for fun (yes, we have actually seen this—or the results of it), and opening other items, such as bags and packages, with your mouth have the potential to loosen teeth, cause chips, cracks, or breaks, or pull out fillings. When outside forces damage your teeth, they encourage bacteria to form in these newly exposed places and weaken tooth structure.

Bruxism—the involuntary or habitual grinding or clenching of the jaw and teeth, often during sleep—also can cause jaw disorders, headaches, earaches, and damaged teeth. Your dentist can intervene by fitting you with an occlusal guard to wear at night. This special cushion can prevent (or mitigate, if issues have already started) problems and pain caused by grinding and/or clenching your teeth while you sleep.

Dental cleanings: How often?

In Chapter 2, we talked about the old Ipana toothpaste campaign featuring "brusha brusha brusha" pitchman Bucky Beaver. The manufacturer, Bristol-Myers, promoted the concept that people should see a dentist every six months for a check-up and cleaning.

But dental cleanings are as individual as you are. The frequency of your check-ups should be determined by your dentist and dental hygienist. As we've discussed, there are people for whom genetics play a huge and favorable role, where they can roll the dice and go years without a cleaning (which we do not recommend!) and not suffer the consequences. For others, as diligent as they are in the care of their teeth, their genetic makeup may work against them, and even six months can be too long to wait between professional cleanings.

Bacteria typically form a film like plastic wrap around the teeth every twenty-four to forty-eight hours that sticks to the tooth's surface and to tissue beneath the gum line, needing to be brushed away—though we hope people are not waiting forty-eight hours to brush! But some people don't brush properly, or even if they do, their brush can't reach the tissue below the gum line. Mouth bacteria may continue to grow, and as the bacteria population gets larger in those dental pockets, it builds up like barnacles on a boat. Plaque accumulation can cause irritation and inflammation to the tissues surrounding the teeth (almost like a splinter).

Once that population of bacteria grows stronger, the toxins it produces start to destroy the bone and surrounding structures around the teeth, weakening the foundation that holds them in their position. When weakened and lost, a domino effect leading to tooth loss will occur. You want to be sure you're getting professional dental cleanings often enough to prevent that from happening.

The cost of clean

We know that where cost is a concern, many patients—especially those without dental insurance—find it challenging to come in every few months for a dental cleaning. Even if they have insurance, cleanings may be covered less often than we recommend, which again depends on the patient's individual oral health. But ignoring the need for cleaning your teeth can cause periodontal disease, a bacterial infection that can be stabilized but not eradicated.

Once you have been diagnosed with periodontal disease, you'll need appropriate therapy, and the condition will need to be tracked, monitored, and readdressed if necessary. As our immune systems wax and wane, our susceptibility to bacterial and viral infections also rises and falls, so gum disease can flare up again, even after successful treatment.

If more frequent professional cleanings are warranted, sometimes it's easier to put another visit or two in perspective by asking yourself how many massages you get a year, or maybe how many visits you make to the chiropractor. Consider the cost of that expensive gym membership (though we certainly do not advocate eliminating exercise), or trips to the nail and hair salon. Keeping your teeth clean will reduce the chance for bacteria to take over, causing periodontal disease and other problems that can amount to many thousands of dollars. From that perspective, getting dental care at the recommended intervals really is a small price to pay. It's part of being your own best dentist—a savvy preemptive strike to protect your health, just like exercise. Regular dental care is part of healthy living.

Got milk? Guess what?

There's a lot of misinformation out there about what to eat—and what not to eat—to help ensure strong teeth. The question of calcium comes up on occasion. Many people are under the misconception—usually because they've seen advertising by the dairy industry—that strong bones and teeth are dependent on the amount of calcium in the body. The fact is, though some research seems to connect the two, we've never seen a scientific study that says ingesting calcium will have a direct impact on tooth health.

Calcium can be found in many non-dairy foods, including vegetables and fruit, as well as obtained from supplements. While we don't recommend ignoring the body's need for this mineral, as far as counting on it to ensure optimal tooth health and prevent tooth loss as we age, we believe there are other factors—which are explored throughout this book—that are far more important.

At the same time, there have been studies showing calcium might have an effect on periodontal disease—which is really an inflammatory response to bacterial products found in dental plaque. Periodontal disease can affect the supporting structures of the teeth.6 Someone deficient in calcium (and/

---

6   Riva Rouger-Decker and Cor van Loveren. "Sugars and dental caries," *The American Journal of Clinical Nutrition* Vol. 78, No. 4 (2003).

or folate and Vitamin C) can have issues with wound healing and inflammatory response, so getting the right amount of all necessary vitamins and minerals—including calcium—is an important part of dental health and overall health.

Acids can erode dental enamel. While we can stay away from constantly drinking acidic sports drinks and soft drinks, and even some bottled waters that contain fruit juice or flavorings from juice, we can't eliminate acidic foods altogether. So many of our important sources of vitamins and minerals come from citrus and other fruits and vegetables, not to mention the pleasure we get from biting into a sweet, juicy orange. To help protect your teeth, take the extra step of following consumption of a high acidity food by doing something as simple as drinking a glass of water, chewing sugarless gum, or brushing your teeth, if possible. This creates the critical buffering effect that helps prevent acid from causing tooth erosion, and eventually periodontal disease and dental decay.

Want to be your own best dentist? Develop good oral care habits, pay attention to your diet, and don't use your teeth for anything other than what they were intended for. Keep your dental appointments. If you practice these habits consistently, they will help you and your dentist form a powerful alliance for a lifetime of care.

http://ajcn.nutrition.org/content/78/4/881S.full

Chapter 6

Can You Always Trust Your Dentist?

Corporate dentistry means dentists don't always practice the way they want

"Who's running the show?" In the world of entertainment, some of the great comedy legends used to utter that famous line. It always produced a laugh amidst chaos and confusion. But the quality of your dental work and thoroughness of your dentist is no laughing matter. Knowing exactly who's in charge can be a critical factor in trusting the treatment you're getting, the quality and longevity of your dental work, and so much more.

In this regard, there is a vast difference between what a private dental practice provides and what corporate dentistry offers. This may include the dentist's level of experience and ability to provide short- and long-term care, as well as the quality of materials used in procedures and the standards and reliability of labs from which they are sourced. Perhaps most important, it can affect the true concern and caring you expect from a dentist and team. Though some patients may see corporate dentistry as a less expensive means to an end, largely due to the volumes of people these business models serve and the cost-cutting measures transferred to them, the result may not always be what you had envisioned.

Of course, it is possible to find wonderful, caring, skilled dentists in private practice *and* in the corporate environment. It is, however, more common to find a dentist most suitable for advanced adult dental needs *and* who provides stellar service in private practice, rather than in a cookie-cutter corporate dental practice. In this chapter, we will discuss the differences and which type of dental practice may be more appropriate for you.

May I take your order?

In corporate dentistry practices—which began to dot the dental landscape about twenty years ago and have grown tremendously—dentists are not owners but rather employees. Though there are exceptions, as employees, they might be less invested in the outcome and long-term effects of the work performed. We all know that sometimes it's easier to write things off and not worry as much about customer service or what happens down the road if we don't *own* something—if our name isn't on it. It's just human nature.

On the other hand, when someone's livelihood and reputation—and the practice's viability and longevity—are based on everything that goes on in their dental chairs every day, the practice may function at a higher level because the dentist feels more accountable. In private practice, the incentive may also be there for the dentist to get to know the patient as a whole individual, including dental history, lifestyle, financial considerations, and long-term goals. This information lets the dentist create a treatment plan in which patient and dentist will be oral health partners for the long haul.

Corporate dentistry became big business when it was realized just how profitable dentistry could be if large volumes of patients could be seen in rapid succession. Some of these enterprises were owned by dentists who developed the concept and then sold it. The groups that took them over—generally individuals who had no background in dentistry—foresaw a successful business model if costs could be reduced and patients of private practices could be lured by lower fees and more convenient hours and appointments.

By partnering with dental suppliers and laboratories (in and outside of the United States), and buying in bulk volume, these corporate practices have been able to reduce their costs significantly compared to a private practice. Also, these large corporate practices decided they would need a much less expensive labor force in order to make as much money as possible. They search for dentists who are recently graduated and are in need of a job to gain experience, as well as dentists who have come from foreign countries looking for work. Often, these individuals are concerned about making money just to pay their bills (as we said in Chapter 3, the average dentist now graduates from dental school with an average of $400,000 in student loan debt). These less-experienced dentists may not yet have been able to get a position in a private practice.

You are more likely to find a "rookie" team employed in corporate enterprises. Seasoned dental hygienists, clinical assistants, and business team members tend to be more inclined to work in practices where the dentist or dentists—and not the corporation—run the show. They know that there is generally greater focus on patients in these private practices and less focus on profits.

Again, to be clear, this does not mean that a dentist working in corporate dentistry is uncaring or without any skill. For many patients, the corporate type of practice and a less-experienced dentist may work out just fine. But we wrote this book with Baby Boomers and an aging population in mind. If you are over age fifty or have multiple dental issues, or just need more TLC, the corporate dentistry model might not meet your expectations.

Everyone has to start somewhere, and in fact, when we were just out of school, we worked for a group practice managed by a corporation. Because we have been dentists in both corporate and private dental practice, we feel qualified to discuss the pros and cons of each. Though we probably had more freedom to diagnose problems and determine treatment plans than many dentists have in a corporate practice setting, we still had quotas to fill (a certain number of this or that procedure to do in order to turn a profit). That's the reason we know this information from the inside out. As we've said before, when all you have in your tool belt is a hammer, everything looks like a nail.

If you go to a restaurant and you're on a limited diet or with a desire for something specific—a dish prepared a certain way that is not on the menu, tailored to your needs and wants—

depending on the establishment's rules, you may or may not be able to get it. It's the same in corporate dentistry. Again, not all corporate dental practices are run poorly and/or with constraints, but many are. Because it's a numbers game—patients in and out, and number and types of procedures recommended, or even mandated for the bottom line—dentists in corporate practices may be somewhat restricted about the level of care they feel they can provide.

Après school

So much of what we learned about the fine art of practicing dentistry occurred after dental school. It's impossible to list all the subtle factors that can have a deep impact on the procedures we recommend to each patient. A large part of what we do in private practice involves looking at individuals from a holistic perspective—their lifestyles and oral health practices—and not just the fact that two weeks' worth of pain brought them in, so maybe they need a root canal. We're going to take the time to look carefully at their entire medical and dental history, ask appropriate questions, collect diagnostic data, and develop a diagnosis. Sometimes this takes time—and time is usually extremely limited in a corporate practice.

In the same situation, a dentist working in corporate dentistry may have a quota of patients to see that day, may feel pressured to meet it, and consequently may not have the time to get to the crux of the problem. In those scenarios, if the source of pain is undetermined or unclear, patients are often referred out to specialists, where they will end up spending even more money and taking more of their time away from work. Anything that doesn't fit the corporate model is considered an inconvenience that needs to be removed from the system. Sometimes, the lack of advanced diagnostic tools creates this kind of scenario, too.

Raising our flag

When the corporation-managed practice for which we worked was bought out by a dental insurance company, we took it as a cue to get out and start our own practice. It became clear that the insurance company only wanted to make money. In fact, within a short time, we were given ultimatums that we considered borderline malpractice. We were strongly encouraged to only provide cheaper, short-term options for patients. Dentistry that cost more and lasted longer took more time and produced less revenue for the practice. Needless to say, that didn't sit well with us. This money-focused strategy turns patients into inanimate commodities instead of flesh-and-blood entities with brains, lifestyles, histories, and plans.

In Chapter 2, we talked about our new patients—some with fears that have kept them away from a dental office for years—and how hard we work to individualize their visits and treatments as well as to develop a relationship with them. In corporate dentistry, there is also a model for running new patients through the office. Patients come in, get their teeth cleaned, have some x-rays, and the dentist may see them quickly and glance at their x-rays—but if they don't have a problem, the dentist doesn't spend as much time with them. In short, they're looking more at the mouth than the person.

In a practice like ours, we're taking all the time necessary to build a relationship, which is more important to us than just the mouth. How can we get to know folks better in order to help them make key decisions about their teeth? How well can we get to know our patients to customize treatment for each and every one of them? Those are our objectives and goals.

In a corporate environment, someone may tell the patient what they need or what they think they need (again, there might be a limited number of procedures they can perform, and they're going to try to fit the patient into one mold or another). There isn't a lot of room for creativity or alternative options. Also, some corporate models offer the dentist commissions if they can sell the patient on certain procedures. Consequently, there may be a conflict between what actually needs to be done and the pressure on the dentist to sell. The dentist might be involved in what is known in retail as "upselling"—convincing the patient to opt for additional or more expensive procedures.

In corporate dentistry, patients may be less involved in decisions about their care than they would be if they saw a dentist in private practice, where typically, the patient is the one in the driver's seat —or at least functioning as the co-pilot. In private practice, the patient and dentist form much more of a partnership.

Where your health is concerned, partnership is important. Having a dentist you can trust, who will take the time to develop that relationship over time, is valuable to many people—especially as we get older and oral health may become more complicated. Having access to a particular dentist, one who knows you, can make a big difference—and in a corporate practice, this is increasingly difficult. Because of the business model of corporate dentistry, dentists tend not to stick around long, so patients get passed from dentist to dentist, This is a concern we hear frequently when we see patients who come from these types of practices.

In our practice, although there may be two or even three dentists involved with a patient's care, there is always a primary dentist. The primary dentist usually sees that patient most frequently and keeps track of their care. When a dentist leaves a corporate practice, many times, the patient has to start all over again with someone new.

Again, it's important to acknowledge that we're using a wide brush to paint a big picture of corporate dentistry, and there are always exceptions. But if a patient develops needs outside the typical cleaning/cavity filling/six-month checkup paradigm, all too often, those needs exceed corporate dentistry's reach.

Picture a house in a development—especially popular in the 1950s and 60s—where rows and rows of residences look alike. Everywhere you look, there is a house just like yours. You can live in the house and still be comfortable, and, in fact, the arrangement might be just fine if you have no problem fitting yourself to the mold. But some people desire a more custom-built environment. There are certain things on which they're not willing to compromise. You will get a much more customized experience when you're a patient in a private dental practice.

The cost of not doing it right the first time

When it comes to affordability, consider the cost of your dental care long-term—not just the cost of a particular service or insurance code. How long will the dental procedure you've just had last? Where were the dental products or restorations made—in a third-world country, in order to cut costs? Or were only the highest quality products and materials used because the dentist guarantees his or her work and wants it to last as long as it can? You can save enormous amounts of money by having a plan. You can avoid potentially expensive dental treatments by having a dentist who can coach you on where to be proactive.

Finally, the dental insurance conundrum is definitely worth mentioning here. Although dental insurance can be utilized and maximized in a corporate dental practice as well as a private practice, there are some differences. In a corporate practice, they often have multiple locations and can bargain for reimbursement increases that would put smaller, private practices out of business. This often means that the private dentist may practice "out of network," while the corporate practice itself is considered a "preferred provider."

Many insurance carriers mandate that their preferred providers meet certain criteria, and these criteria are never about dentists' credentials or the quality of care they perform. The only thing the insurance companies want is to come to an agreement on fees. Insurance companies basically bargain with dentists to lower their usual and customary fees. In return, the insurance company will refer patients to them by putting their name on a list of preferred providers. That might sound like a good deal for the patient—but not always.

Dentists have to make up the money from reduced fees somehow. How do they do it? Maybe they use a less expensive lab, work faster in order to see more patients, and/or "sell" more dentistry. While there are plenty of dentists with good intentions who are also signed up as preferred providers, the pressure to make up a deficit in fees can be enormous. Most, if not all, dentists would prefer not to do this, but they might see it as a necessary evil to keep patients coming through the door.

Many dentists believe that if the insurance company doesn't refer patients, they will have a difficult time finding them. These dentists essentially are held hostage by the insurance companies. The insurers often exploit their preferred dentists by taking months to reimburse them for the work they have done. Feelings of frustration and discontent with the insurance companies that essentially "own" these dentists are rampant. The inherent caveat is this: if dentists know they have to give you a significant discount—and might not receive payment from the insurance company for an extended period of time— will they treat you any differently than they treat their patients who do not have insurance and subsequently are not part of this exasperating scenario?

Our practice operates with the opposite perspective, aiming to offer the highest quality treatment options and service to all patients, whether they have dental insurance or not. Clearly, we're not alone in our philosophy, and we are grateful there are other practices out there that work this way as well. Because we have never agreed to a contract with the insurance companies, we can also act as a mediator for our patients in the event an insurance company decides to deny benefits for any reason. Preferred providers generally waive this right in their contracts, so if patients are denied benefits, they are on their own.

Many patients don't know that an out-of-network dentist can still maximize a patient's dental benefits and get them the reimbursement to which their insurance company has agreed. The insurance companies don't want you to know that, because they will have to pay out a higher amount of benefit than they would if you went to one of their preferred providers—which means less money for the insurance company. They also have to pay the claim faster, which prevents them from accruing more interest from the bank. Thankfully there have been state laws passed that prevent insurance companies from holding onto patient benefits longer than thirty days (at least here in North Carolina) as long as the assignment of benefits goes directly to the policy holder.

Does this mean that you should always seek an out-of-network dentist? Not necessarily. We would never suggest that out-of-network dentists are more qualified or caring than dentists who are considered in-network. Just make sure you choose your dentist using a lot of criteria, as expressed throughout this book. Don't make your choice based solely on how they file your dental insurance.

The decision is yours. Like many things, dentistry is not a one-size-fits-all proposition. We encourage patients to do their research and find out as much information as possible about a practice going in. Don't wait until after a visit or procedure, when it may be too late.

Chapter 7

Customizing Care to Your Needs and Circumstances

Dental procedures are the "new black"!

n dentistry, the words "always" and "never" don't exist. What we mean is, there are many factors that can go into making a decision about what kind of procedure is best for you. To that end, we do not "always" do certain things or "never" do other things.

Treatment is as customized and unique as each individual who walks into the office, which, as far as we are concerned, is the only way to practice dentistry. What makes sense for one person absolutely may not make sense for another who appears to be in a similar position. It may not make sense aesthetically, socially, emotionally, in the realm of managing pain, or economically. Everyone's goals for his or her teeth are different.

In diagnosing a problem and arriving at the best solution, that partnership between you and your dentist that we've emphasized in previous chapters is essential. When you are confident the dentist is listening to you and looking out for your best interests, you are on the right path. Great dentists will listen first and then determine, with your input, what your best options might be. If they have the skill set for that option, they will charge you a fair price for their services. If they lack a certain skill set, dentists of this caliber will know their limitations and help you find another dentist or specialist who can ensure the most appropriate outcome.

The best dentists understand that running a profitable business is important. They know they need to hire the best people and use technology that makes a patient's life more comfortable as they keep their dentistry of the highest quality. All this can be achieved by keeping fees fair and reasonable and running the business efficiently.

A few years ago, we had a patient come through the door who had spent $40,000 rebuilding her mouth with another dentist. She'd wanted veneers, dental implants, and more, and the dentist had complied—sort of. But the other dentist was clearly practicing above the level of his skill set, and it had ended badly for her. The work had been done improperly and had begun breaking down two years after it was completed.

This patient had made the rounds of five dental offices before coming to us. Each new dentist she saw acknowledged the damage but said they weren't sure they could do anything to fix it. They recommended that, at the very least, she seek legal recourse from the original dentist. We told her we could help her, but it would likely cost another $40,000 or more to fix it all. It's much harder to clean up someone else's mistakes than to start from scratch.

She returned a year later, ready to embark on her new journey. In a very frank discussion, with aesthetics also on the table, I asked her if she didn't want to ever worry again about having another tooth break, or needing a root canal, or a cap issue, or a bridge falling out. She replied—with tears in her eyes and a broken voice—that yes, all of that was what she truly wanted. In fact, the reason she had sought such extensive care from the dentist who ended up doing all the damage was her lifetime of dental frustration from cavities, gum disease, and broken teeth. As we've said before, genetics can play a huge role in oral health. Unfortunately, she'd not been dealt a good hand.

Because she wanted a mouth that consistently looked good, one that enabled her to chew her food without issue and would not produce any more surprises or pain—not even so much as a toothache—it was clear that dental implants were the right course of action for her.

"Let's consider rebuilding your mouth by starting with a clean slate. By removing the organic structures (the teeth) and placing inert titanium dental implants, we will have a foundation you can count on," I told her. She basically was going to have a "bionic mouth"! For all intents and purposes, it would be impervious to pain and bacterial or acid destruction.

After she spoke to the rest of our surgical team, she felt 100 percent certain this was the right choice. It took some time, but we planned it out and did all the work. While she still needs to maintain her new dental implants with regular dental cleanings, the prognosis is excellent. She will have none of the previous frustrations she had suffered through—instead, she can look forward to a consistently beautiful smile.

Baby Boomers benefit!

Practices like ours are a bit of a new phenomenon. We primarily focus on the needs of a more mature demographic. Our typical patient is a Baby Boomer in his or her fifties, sixties, or seventies, though we treat older patients. We have structured our practice to meet the needs of a subset of the population that suffered through earlier days of dentistry. Most of our patients have old metal fillings that are failing, missing, and/or broken, and they have discolored teeth. Many have spent a lot of money trying to keep up with their dental needs but have lost confidence or are confused by new procedures that may have been recommended to them.

It is not uncommon for patients in our practice to have a significant fear of having dental work done, being unhappy with the appearance of their smile, or not being able to chew the foods they love. In order to focus on the needs of adults, it's important that practices like ours pay more attention to developing trust and properly diagnosing problems, with less emphasis on "drill and fill," children's dentistry, or volume-based, dental-mill procedures.

When considering dental options and trying to make a financially responsible decision, we like to use the analogy of walking through doors. If the number of steps or procedures that must be done to save a tooth, for example—let's call it Door Number One—far exceed the benefit and/or cost of extracting that tooth and replacing it with a dental implant (which is as good as or better than a natural tooth)—call it Door Number Two— we usually recommend the latter.

One of the biggest issues we see is where people have been told they need to have all their teeth removed—with no discussion and no other options given. There should ALWAYS be a discussion because there are so many alternatives out there. Fortunately, most patients have the good sense to get another opinion. Or maybe they've been trying to save teeth, one by one, and their previous dentist wasn't looking at the big picture. Perhaps it really was in the patient's best interest to explore options that might include removing some or all of the teeth and finding solutions that are less dependent on bacterial levels, mouth acidity, and force issues. Some individuals cannot live with the idea of a denture, while others can't live without it.

Some people have the notion that only their front teeth matter because those are the ones that show. Others only care if they have back teeth so they can chew. One gentleman told us he didn't care what his smile looked like; his wife was the only one who was going to see it anyway. We proposed to him that his front teeth do matter to her, and she is the one who prepares his meals, so he'd better make sure she loves his smile!

In reality, both front and back teeth are important, for different reasons. What is most important in adult dentistry is looking at the mouth as a complex organ, and not just homing in on one tooth and missing the big picture. Customizing care is an ever-evolving, multi-faceted kind of process, often with changing priorities. The best dentists understand that and will find ways to help you fit dentistry into your budget and lifestyle.

The following are some examples of people whose lives were affected in a big way, and for the better, by customized dental care.

Sal

While we first met him in Chapter 2, it's important to emphasize here that one of our patients was a heavy smoker who didn't like what had happened to his teeth. In fact, it's fair to say that he had a real aversion to dentistry and dental care. His gums were receding quite far, his teeth appeared jumbled and discolored, and he had a lot of pain and discomfort. Because he traveled internationally for his job, he wanted his teeth pulled so he'd not be stuck dealing with dental problems that might come up while he was far from home, without a dentist he knew and trusted—perhaps one who barely spoke English! We assessed the situation and determined he probably had a couple more years left before he'd have to do anything as drastic as total mouth extractions. But he'd reached the conclusion himself that now was the time.

We explored dental implants, which can be done different ways. We specifically looked at an implant hybrid restoration, which has a very strong zirconium, titanium, or synthetic fiber reinforced framework and nano ceramic restorations on top of the framework that look as close to natural teeth as possible. Our patient said, "I want the best," and while this is not typical of everyone, he had the financial resources to go with this option. His teeth were removed and dental implants were placed in the upper and lower jaws.

Sal went through the process of wearing a temporary acrylic prosthesis during the healing and integration part of the process. We used that time to evaluate his aesthetics and even changed the design to mimic slight crowding of the lower teeth, to simulate a more natural appearance. After the integration time was over and we were ready to convert to his final prosthesis, he was thrilled to finally get his new smile tightened down and in place. In fact he could barely contain his excitement on the day of delivery.

Sal walked out of our office a new man with a spring to his step as he smiled from ear to ear at everyone. As we said in Chapter 2, in the end, he joked with us that while expensive, it was worth it to be pain free with a perfect smile. And now that perfect smile could help close million-dollar deals—in any language! He calls it the best decision he's ever made, and he reminds us of that whenever he comes in for a cleaning.

Monica

Monica's story is different, though not out of step with some the patients who come to our office believing there is only way to solve a problem. Because of the breadth and scope of the customized care we provide, educating patients is an integral part of our practice. Monica provided us with another opportunity to do that.

Her concern was that she had been told her teeth were crooked and yellow. By conventional standards, we didn't think it was much of an issue; in fact, her teeth looked quite pretty, and maybe just a tad crooked. But because she'd been told by family members that her teeth were not straight and was self-conscious about them, we wanted to present her with all the options. At her first appointment, she brought up porcelain veneers, which are often the right choice for teeth that are not straight or are discolored. But in Monica's case, veneers would have been a more invasive and expensive approach to fixing a problem that could be easily accomplished with a different method.

The alternative in this case included a far less costly procedure called Six Month Smiles™, a short-term orthodontic program that straightens teeth within four to six months, in addition to KoR Whitening™. We used computer technology to show her the magic of cosmetic imagery, and Monica was delighted with the results on the screen. She elected to do it. In our practice we call this "value engineering"—saving the patient potentially thousands of dollars with equally effective results. Unfortunately, not all dentists will take the time to apprise patients of alternatives, although some might.

Had Monica gone somewhere else, there's a possibility she may have ended up enduring a lengthy, invasive procedure and perhaps parting with a large sum of money she didn't need to spend. When we got right down to it, there was a better plan we were able to customize for her that provided a more natural outcome and didn't break the bank.

Monica only wanted straight, white teeth. She didn't particularly want dental veneers, but she had thought that porcelain veneers were the only option. Good dentists will not make recommendations for a specific treatment until they know what you want to accomplish. The more you can tell your dentist about your expectations, the better he or she will be able to help you find the options that work just for you.

Patti

When Patti came to us, she was resigned to the burgeoning crow's feet developing around her eyes and also the lines and drooping around her mouth. She felt prematurely old. Her opening statement was, "I have an old-lady smile, and with this much energy and 'va-va-voom,' I need my smile to match it!"

While we do not profess to be dermatologists or plastic surgeons, there are ways we can improve someone's outward appearance by transforming a worn-out and worn-down smile. Too many people don't realize that with the right dental procedure, a smile that is sadly lacking in the right number of teeth showing, or has worn edges, can be transformed into a bright, youthful, uplifted, and engaging smile that can take years off the appearance of someone's teeth and face.

As we age, we wear our teeth down, which ages the way we look—sometimes prematurely. That youthful smile can fade without firm lip support. For example, when teeth are removed during the preparation for dentures, the patient's bone and soft tissue can start to recede, because they have no support. This causes that "puckered" look that is evident when dentures are taken out for the night. Dentures that replace a whole mouthful of teeth are only plastic, and eventually they wear down, too—even faster than natural teeth, because of the nature of the material. So what once was the solution for replacing all the teeth initially is no longer serving its purpose. In fact, it is detracting and becoming more of a nuisance than a solution. As further bone absorption occurs, dentures don't fit as well and can slip, causing areas of the mouth to become sore as they chew and function.

Once this happens, the patient starts trying to find out which dental adhesive holds the longest—the one that won't start slipping after three hours or the one that will last as long as the package says it will. Some patients tell us they have "tried every adhesive on the market" and nothing has worked to their satisfaction. Additionally, it can be a challenge to remove all that goop stuck to their dentures and mouth so they can repeat the process the next day. The frustration of not having something dependable and comfortable to wear, combined with compromised aesthetics, in time leaves the wearer feeling like a hostage to dentures, even though the purpose of getting dentures is to make life easier.

You might be wondering what happened to Patti. Once we discussed what her desires were and what we could do for her, the final outcome included lower porcelain restorations and a new upper denture plate. She had looked and felt older than she was, partly because her former ten-teeth replacement appliance barely showed when she smiled. The teeth were very small for her face. The combined wear of her natural teeth and her replacement teeth positioned her jaw, and consequently her facial features, in such a way that they made her mouth appear sunken and older.

We picked a lighter shade of teeth and selected a tooth shape that fit her facial features. The surfaces of both her natural teeth and her new denture teeth were set in such a way that it elongated her face, smoothing out the lines and wrinkles around her mouth. This instantly gave her a more youthful and beautiful smile. Patti was ecstatic, exclaiming, "Now my smile matches just how young I feel!"

* * *

Very recently, a new patient—age seventy—came to us as a result of one of our dental implant seminars. He believed he needed all of his teeth extracted. He said he'd been very distressed when another dentist (or actually more than one) had told him that, if he didn't get his teeth removed, he would not be able to eat. Though he now understood the merits of implants, a full mouth extraction was the last thing he ever wanted to go through. An examination showed he had many healthy teeth and no evidence of cavities. He had a few failing dental restorations, some back teeth missing on the lower right side, and about a 50 percent bone loss. He was adamant about not wearing dentures.

In respect to his ideas about himself, our treatment plan definitely did not include a full mouth extraction. In fact, we never believed it was warranted. We presented a plan to him for dental implants on the lower right, with a fixed bridge and a couple of caps. He also needed some periodontal care. If he commits to maintaining the work we do, taking good care of the rest of his natural teeth and seeing us every three to six months, he should be able to keep his teeth for the rest of his life. That's what he wanted. Rather than taking out all his teeth, we were able to accommodate him without reservation.

So what's important to you? Whatever goals you may have that include the brightest, healthiest smile ever, customizing care to your needs and circumstances is among the things we do best—and about which we're the most excited!

Chapter 8
The Joy of Dental Implants

Having your cake and eating it too!

S ometimes we don't realize how much better life can be with a few important fixes, such as having a beautiful, durable, functional mouth. And with proper care, your teeth can last decades—even to the end of your life. After years of pain, discomfort, expense, and the inconvenience many people experience from problems with their natural teeth and gums, who wouldn't want to look and feel great? Dental implants can make that happen.

First, the stats:

- In adults ages thirty-five to forty-four, 69 percent have lost at least one tooth.
- By age seventy-four, 26 percent of adults have lost all of their teeth.
- An estimated thirty million people in the United States have no teeth. Most of them have limited options when it comes to what they can eat, such as an unhealthy diet of soft, starchy foods.

People often experience 40 to 50 percent ridge (bone) loss only six months after losing teeth—and that bone loss is irreversible. With missing teeth, without the root or an implant in place, the jawbone can shrink, making the face look older. Bone loss affects the way we look and feel and can also result in nerve pain.

Dentures and partial dentures only afford 50 percent of natural bite force, resulting in reduced chewing efficiency and subsequent digestive issues. When dentures fit poorly—which can happen as we age—facial structure can change, if we don't keep up with regular maintenance and realignments. Structural changes only compound these problems. So why do we lose our teeth?

We lose them as a result of tooth decay or cavities—which can even form under old dental work. Root canal failure also can cause tooth loss, as can periodontal disease—the most common reason adults lose their teeth. Trauma to the mouth—such as sailing over the handlebars of a bicycle face-first (Chapter 2 adventure!)—can cause tooth loss, as can congenital defects such as weak teeth, soft teeth, and less density to the enamel, which we've covered. Overall dental "wear and tear," which can happen with age—no matter how we take care of our teeth—is another reason. And it's important to note that when teeth are missing, if there is no root or an implant in place, the jawbone can shrink, making the face look older.

If you opt for dentures, understand that they are acrylic teeth and gums that fit over the ridges of your mouth. It's easier to keep an upper plate in place on the roof of the mouth, with the help of oral adhesives, but adhesives can be unreliable. It's often very difficult to keep bottom dentures in place because they don't have the benefit of suction; and even with adhesives, and the tongue and muscles of the mouth are constantly battling this chunky, acrylic object. In short, dentures tend to be uncomfortable and hard to wear. They don't stay in place when you chew. Loose-fitting dentures can affect speech and restrict your food options.

People with dentures often lack confidence in their appearance and worry about the stigma attached to them. Some of our more courageous patients have admitted to us that their dentures significantly restrict the enjoyment of particular intimate social experiences they used to enjoy. Dentures are a handicapping kind of prosthesis, and they have been for years. There has been little change in the design evolution and subsequent wearer-friendly component of dentures. However, within the last ten years or so, new options have begun to evolve for individuals trapped in dentures.

Warning: Bone loss!

After giving lectures on dental implants for many years to the public and prospective patients, we have come to realize that there is something that very few individuals with missing teeth realize. It has become the take-away from our lectures and something that patients who attend always bring up afterwards. You must understand this as well, as it will directly affect what options you may or may not have after a tooth is removed. Bone loss ALWAYS occurs after a tooth is removed from your jaw. The more teeth you have removed, the greater the bone loss. The longer the period of time a jaw is without teeth, the more bone disappears.

Ask most people who have worn dentures for years to remove their teeth and you will see their faces "cave in," so to speak. This is all because of the loss of supporting bone in the jaws. Now, not only the mouth is affected, but the face. And this kind of bone loss is impossible to reverse. There are ways we can graft bone into the mouth, but in the later stages, this procedure can be terribly invasive and unpredictable—not to mention expensive. The longer a person waits to replace a missing tooth or teeth, the more invasive and expensive it can be to fix the problem.

If you are one of these people who have a significant amount of bone loss already, do not lose hope. Advancements in technology are making it easier for us to help you.

What about dental implants?

The most exciting new development was the invention of dental implants, which can be used to replace teeth. Implants can help in two ways. With a titanium screw as a base, the implant is set into the bone—essentially replacing the root— and can act as an anchor for a single tooth or multiple teeth. The dental implant supports an abutment, which is a cylinder that screws into it. Then a crown or a different type of appliance can be attached to the abutment. Dental implants can also be used as a retention device to hold a special kind of denture (not to be confused with conventional dentures, which have no anchor) in place.

A single crown or cap can be screwed down or cemented to an implant; a ring of teeth—up to fourteen teeth in all—can be screwed down to four implants if we are rebuilding someone's mouth. A dental implant mirrors the design, structure, and function of a normal tooth and becomes the strongest "tooth" in your mouth. The implant, which goes into the jawbone and holds the abutment base and crown in place, is made of titanium—a material highly biocompatible with bone. Titanium is commonly used in joint replacement, as at the hip, shoulder, and knee. Dental implants immediately stop bone loss, preclude further tooth decay and gum disease, and are a highly secure, usually permanent option. They are designed to be yours for life.

Many of our patients come to us having worn conventional dentures for five or ten years or more. Frankly, they've had enough. They've labored over preparing their prosthetic teeth every day and dealing with goopy, stringy, foul-tasting adhesives that may not always work. They've struggled to keep the plates in while they eat the way they should be able to, and they have worn down the artificial teeth. Traditional dentures often thin out and crack, so every few years they should be replaced or, at the very least, relined and balanced. At the same time, as the dentures are wearing down, the patient's nose-to-chin ratio gets shorter. At some point, rather than investing more money in the same impermanent process, many people tend to opt for a new look and a better way.

Bang for your buck

At our practice, as we have mentioned previously, we are big on "value engineering." This means getting the most value for your dollar and finding creative ways to keep patients from having to waste their money in the future. Dental implants are more affordable than they have ever been, and sometimes if a patient already has a set of dentures, we can place a few implants, for example, to provide stability on the bottom where traditional dentures fail. This procedure improves their capability to eat and, more importantly to some, offers a sense of security that the teeth will stay in place. It is also one of the most cost-effective uses of dental implants.

Though some dentures can be retrofitted to an overdenture (especially if they've been made in the last couple of years), many people will need a new appliance made, whether it's an overdenture, a hybrid-type screw-down appliance, or something else along those lines. For individuals without teeth who keep putting off the process and are living with loose or ill-fitting dentures, the options for dental implants can dwindle. The costs of delay include the need for bone grafting, a sinus lift, or—in extreme cases—a combination of the two. In essence, the longer you wait, the more expensive the solutions may become.

Knowledge plus reputation equals results

While there is no recognized specialty in dental implants, education and experience are the best teachers. Try to find a dentist who has both of these and has earned a reputation for success. Understanding the multitude of products and applications of state-of-the-art equipment and technology is of key importance in a successful outcome.

Every patient who has a dental implant wants a successful outcome. The reality is that most dental implants placed (up to 98 percent in studies) are successful. However, a number of implants fail, and that number tends to be higher in the hands of an unskilled or undereducated practitioner. If you do your research, you will find that some common reasons dental implants fail are variables that are directly related to the patient's body or health.

What is less commonly discussed is implant failure caused by the lack of experience and judgment on the part of the dentist. He must take certain precautions, such as properly preparing the implant site; using the appropriate implant size, type or design for the site; placing the implant at the right location and the right angle; avoiding nerves and other potential anatomical obstacles; and not applying excessive loads or balancing forces. If the dentist doesn't do all these things, problems can result, and implant failure is imminent.

Who can have dental implants?

Almost everyone is a good candidate for dental implants, but there are exceptions. Certain medications called bisphosphonates, used to treat osteoporosis, may adversely affect the jawbone's ability to break down or remodel itself, which can undermine its healing capacity. While implants are not impossible to attempt when people are on these medications, their side effects can make dental implants risky. If you don't heal well because of a disease such as uncontrolled diabetes mellitus, or if you have an immune system disorder that precludes proper healing, dental implants are generally not recommended. People who have radiation treatments to the head and neck might develop a condition called osteoradionecrosis, meaning they lack the blood vessels in the bone to help them heal. Smokers may also have issues because of the way nicotine constricts capillaries, which means they may not heal well, limiting the odds of a successful outcome for dental implants.

There is a myth, however, that because you reach a certain age, you are not a good candidate for dental implants. Age in itself usually has nothing to do with having the right physical disposition for the procedure, unless you are also compromised by the health issues referenced above. To help determine if someone is a good candidate, a thorough medical and dental history should be completed as well as a complete examination of the head, neck, mouth, and jaws.

A CT scan of the potential implant patient's jaw should be taken, which allows us to see important landmarks such as major nerves and blood vessels, and to judge pathways to place the implants. A traditional x-ray isn't enough; it's a two-dimensional rendering of the jaw, while a CT scan is a three-dimensional rendering. While the former may show cavities and bone height, there's no way for it to determine essential width unless someone goes in surgically, peels back the gums, and measures with a ruler! The CT scan reveals the best location to place the implants and can also give us readings on the density of the bone. If you are considering dental implants you must have a CT or 3D scan taken of the area, in our opinion. Today, these diagnostic films are considered the standard of care. The best implant dentists will have this technology in their practices.

Using the correct-size implant is also imperative. Molars, for example, have different dimensions than other teeth. They are larger, and because they are the so-called "chewing teeth," they play an integral role in keeping other teeth from shifting.

If size is not considered, you could end up with what we call a "tomato on a stick": a titanium post that's quite narrow in diameter with a big, fat tooth on top of it. This can become troublesome to the patient because it can trap food scraps and make gum cleaning difficult.

Another issue would be the general physics of balancing a significantly larger object on top of a smaller one. These problems are headed off at the pass when we use an appropriate implant size. Molars generally require a minimum of a five- to six-millimeter diameter implant, and molar-sized implants can actually go up to nine millimeters in diameter—because the mouth is definitely not a one-size-fits-all proposition!

Placing the implant immediately after the natural tooth is extracted is also advantageous. Getting a dental implant to be "in service"—at the point where the patient can use it confidently and without restriction in the way teeth should function—once took a year. Today, we usually have it down to about three months.

Another key to having successful implants—so that you can rely on a beautiful, functional set of teeth—is implant maintenance. You will still need to go to the dentist for regular cleanings. If you let a lot of plaque and/or biofilm accumulate around the implants, and the gums become irritated and puffy, you might start losing the foundation and support of the bone around the implant.

So if you're healthy and have bones with enough mass (which we determine with a CT scan), and if you are inclined to take the necessary steps to maintain good oral health, you're likely a good candidate for dental implants. If you are missing teeth or have worn dentures and are tired of the hit-or-miss implications of an unstable appliance, dental implants can make your life much better and easier.

Replacement teeth have been around in theory and practice since the time of the ancient Egyptians, more than 3,000 years ago. They used gold, shells, and rocks (ouch!) to replace teeth. Today's dental implants can provide for a lifetime of comfortable, functional usage—and of course, that perfectly enviable smile!

Chapter 9

How Cosmetic Dentistry Builds Self-Esteem

The kinds of patients we see and the problems we solve: physical and emotional

People are often quick to pass judgment on appearances. While the cliché about "not judging a book by its cover" never quite goes away, what isn't taken into account is just how much we judge ourselves by the way we look. Sometimes, we don't even give others a chance to do it. We are all too eager to be critical of our nose or mouth, jaw line, hair, height, weight, body type, and more. Some people are relentlessly self-critical, spending thousands and thousands of dollars on health spas, diet plans, fitness coaches, Botox, fillers, and drastic plastic surgeries.

Cosmetic dentistry can make a surprisingly significant change in your appearance. Not only can it make your teeth look better, but it can help reshape your lips, jaw line, cheeks, and facial dimensions—nearly the entire face—which can take years off your appearance. That's why some people consider it the best-kept secret in improving our looks.

Whenever we hear someone say, "These kinds of things don't bother me. I'm not concerned about my appearance," an alarm goes off. We know that person is concerned, because he or she is the one who brought it up! Such people may have a self-esteem issue with their smiles, which can be proven by simply asking them to smile. Many times, patients like this don't show their teeth. We call it an "uncooperative" smile. It's not a full, unencumbered, uninhibited, big, broad smile—the kind that comes from deep down inside that you just can't suppress. The smile that expresses joy is in there somewhere—unless someone is working hard at hiding his or her teeth.

Sometimes people are looking for permission to get their smiles fixed because a spouse, parent, or other family member or friend has given them the idea that, if they do anything to improve their appearance, they are being vain, selfish—even sinful! While we don't wish to embark on any kind of religious tangent, some might say, if God didn't want us to smile, He'd not have given us the muscles to do so. If you're not happy with your smile, there's absolutely nothing wrong with improving it. There are no points subtracted for doing everything in your power to feel confident and attractive. In fact, the more confidence you have in your smile, the more likely you are to make someone else smile!

The flip side is if you're taking something that looks good already and going all out to make it completely flawless. If you're striving for an unnatural look, you're probably taking it too far. But to want to give yourself a normal, attractive, natural-looking smile is, well, natural! It makes you seem more personable and approachable, in part because that's what you feel and project. A great smile is a welcome mat. It's reassuring. And when you are confident about your looks, the sky's the limit. Just ask people who have gone through life consistently unhappy about their appearance and what happens after they take control and change it.

Transfiguring Tiffany

One of our patients was very attractive, a lover-of-life woman in her fifties—someone who'd spent thousands of dollars on maintaining her face and her whole body. Tiffany (her name has been changed) was clearly aesthetically driven. She wanted a Hollywood smile to match her "out there!" lifestyle. But she had teeth that didn't complement the look she'd been creating with cosmetic surgery. Her smile was definitely on the list, as she desired a bright, white, youthful one.

There was another detail she wanted addressed, if possible. For years, she'd been treated with fillers and Botox to combat the usual lines that appear around the eyes and mouth as we age. Her wish was that, while fixing her teeth, we could "do something about plumping up (her) lips." In fact, she'd said it somewhat in jest, but in reality, by adding more support for her upper lip, using the veneering process, we told her we could actually make it happen.

Surprised as she was at the idea, Tiffany jumped in. We did twelve porcelain veneers on the top and ten on the bottom. After the procedure was done and she was in her temporaries, she was thrilled with her new look. In fact, she asked if we could plump up her lip even further, but we explained that we could only do so much. She would still need some of her enhancement procedures, but certainly not to the same extent as before. More importantly, she had a straight, white, beautiful smile that aligned with her vision of youth and vitality—which made Tiffany even more of a go-getter!

Designing Dixie

Over time, as we age, we can lose length in our teeth or lose the vertical dimension of our teeth. This essentially affects the height of the lower third of your face. Some dentists may only fix a tooth here and there without addressing what happens during aging, as the chin-to-nose ratio gets smaller. Cosmetic dentistry can increase that vertical dimension, taking years off.

One of our patients—a perfectly coiffed and coutured, elegant and exuberant Southern belle whose spirit and vitality would never grow old—had issues relative to the physical aging of her face. She warranted what we call a combination case. She came to our office with worn lower teeth and an upper denture that was not helping her esthetically.

She told us her previous dentist had copied the way her original teeth had looked, even though she had asked him to give her a more youthful look. She felt she looked older than she was, and when she talked, her loose-fitting denture made her slur some words. She also didn't like the fact that the corners of her mouth had been consistently red and cracked since her last plate was made—about six years earlier. We listened and then discussed why she was having those issues. The core of her issues was the vertical dimension of her face.

In the years before her upper plate was made, she'd worn her teeth down to an uneven pattern because her dental issues had been addressed one item at a time. Things were compounded after she had her upper teeth removed and a denture made (to match her worn and uneven lower teeth). Again, time was working against her as she continued to chew and function against her upper denture; the lower teeth were wearing the same pattern into the acrylic teeth in her denture. It was as if the process was repeating itself, but this time at a much faster pace. Her middle face was continuing to shrink because of the further wear of her natural teeth combined with the slow resorption of the bony ridge due to an ill-fitting upper denture.

The solution to her problem was to make her a new upper denture and restore her lower teeth in porcelain to an even surface. Combined, these built up the vertical dimension of her face, which gave her a more youthful look. While correcting years of wear and returning her chewing function to what it once was, we were able to address her aesthetic concerns as well.

In her genteel, Southern way, with a shot of ebullience for good measure, she told us her life had been transformed. Any reticence she'd felt about "putting her best face forward" was gone. This is a great example of how addressing a functional concern can carry with it an aesthetic or cosmetic component that, in the long run, builds the patient's confidence in showing off a smile. We also helped restore her chewing function, improved her speech, and gave her back the dimension in which her facial muscles operate more efficiently.

Transforming Tom

Tom was a sixty-eight-year-old patient who, in the vein we mentioned earlier, was someone who'd professed he was "not at all concerned" with his appearance. Upon asking him to smile, we knew he was deeply concerned, as his smile was more or less forced. As he got older, he admitted, he'd consumed a lot of soft drinks that had eroded the fronts of his teeth. They'd become progressively more yellow and worn down as the enamel was dissolved by these drinks. By his own admission, his smile was not a show-stopper—and now he was having trouble thoroughly chewing food.

The procedure we decided to perform was as much for function as aesthetics. A decision was made to cap each tooth as a protective layer, so he would not lose them, and also to provide a bright new surface that looked more like teeth and less like a patchwork quilt.

It wasn't long before we learned that he was smiling in church and smiling in family photographs. For years, he'd been perceived as stern or distant because he'd been ashamed of revealing his teeth! His new smile was no longer forced. It was completely natural and he couldn't help showing it off to close friends and family. Now Tom has a smile that looks great—and for the rest of his life, his teeth will give him the pleasure of eating the foods he loves.

Reimagining Ronald

In a powerful "don't judge a book by its cover" set of circumstances, Ronald came to our office scruffily unshaven, in rumpled work clothes, and a dirty baseball cap. Although he quickly became one of our favorite patients, at the time, we weren't sure what to make of him. Frankly, we didn't know what he wanted with our office! There was always the possibility he was a contemporary version of Howard Hughes (we later joked with him about that), who paid little attention to his appearance in the last years of his life even though he clearly had the resources for dental services—but we knew that was a long shot!

He asked us to fix his teeth with veneers. Though he began in a lighthearted manner, he became quite serious as he told us he hated his smile. He was discouraged—the condition of his mouth was definitely in his way. We took some x-rays and realized many, if not most, dentists would have turned him away at that point. His teeth were just so jumbled and defaced that not even veneers would have worked to fix them. He needed his entire mouth redone from the bottom up.

When he came back for a second appointment to explore things further, we almost didn't recognize him. He was clean-shaven and nicely dressed. He explained that the last time, he'd come from a job site where he'd been addressing someone's sewer problems. While he wasn't Howard Hughes, Ronald certainly wasn't who he'd appeared to be. He was a hard-working, hands-on businessman. We understood his desire for a better appearance.

"I'm embarrassed to talk to my tenants," he'd told us, "because some of them look like they have more money than I do. They just look nicer." We soon came to know him as a kind, genuine individual with a great sense of humor. We were pleased to be able to help him.

Because his teeth were badly broken down, he understood we were going to have to remove them all and use the bone as a foundation. We did some cosmetic imaging on our computer at no cost—something we like to do for patients—and presented him with the results. When the issue of cost came up, we compared it to a King Ranch—the Mercedes of Ford pick-up trucks, with which we figured he'd be familiar because of his line of work. Turns out he owned one! That was more fuel for the "don't judge a book by its cover" tenet.

We told Ronald the work would include extensive dental implants. Without hesitation, he green-lighted the procedures.

When we had finished, in typical fashion, he produced a Dollar Tree shopping bag full of cash to cover his bill. He also became a willing before-and-after model for some of our advertising, proclaiming that cosmetic dentistry was the best thing he'd ever done for himself, "bar none."

Driving Don (or Don drives us!)

There's no question that everyone wants to look good. Who doesn't want to live in the world as the best version of themselves in every sense of the word: intellectually, emotionally, physically, and aesthetically?

When we first started practicing, we had a patient come into our office like a whirlwind. "You have to help me!" was the first breathless sentence out of his mouth. We couldn't imagine what he was going to say next.

"My teeth are crooked. We've got to get them straight—right away!" he elaborated.

He'd just seen a career consultant who had told him that some people interpret crooked teeth as dishonesty, and he was terrified his customers would see him that way. He was at the beginning of his sales career and rife with ambition. He wanted nothing to stand in his way. He had a lot to prove.

We did a full set of veneers and didn't see Don again for about ten years or maybe longer, at which time he came in for a cleaning. He'd gained about fifty pounds, but his teeth looked fantastic! His sales career was through the roof. He had felt so confident about his totally straight smile when he'd left our office, more a decade earlier, and we know that was a big part of how he presented himself in his business.

The psychological and emotional component of how we see ourselves, and want others to see us, is a big part of how we conduct ourselves in life and what kind of lives develop for us along the way. Brian in Chapter 1 is probably the most compelling example of the merits of cosmetic dentistry. Once his mouth was rebuilt, he rose rapidly through the ranks from a semi-reclusive car washer to a car salesman to dealership finance department manager—with a beautiful family to boot.

Praising Pastor Terry

Perhaps one of the most powerful examples of the work we've done in the area of cosmetic dentistry was a gospel singer and pastor named Terry. Pastor Terry continues to tell us we changed his life.

As a young boy in foster care, Pastor Terry admittedly suffered great abuse and neglect on many levels. He'd also had what he calls a "traumatic" experience with a dentist at a young age, which created a lot of fear in him about ever seeing another one. By the time he was an adult—trying to fulfill his calling in religious songs, videos, and preaching before hundreds of people each week—he'd lost most of his teeth. People's reactions when they saw him hampered his efforts and diminished his confidence in bringing his heartfelt ministry to the world. He'd even considered abandoning his mission.

But after we rebuilt his mouth, he called his new smile "a launching pad for the ministry." He knows he can stand before people unashamed, for the first time in his adult life. He says he smiles incessantly, which makes his words and work far-reaching and much more effective.

Then and now

When cosmetic dentistry first came onto the scene, it was unaffordable for many people. But because of evolving materials, products, procedures, and technology, 21st century cosmetic dentistry is now in a new, affordable realm for most prospective patients. Today, there are some relatively inexpensive procedures we can do to create a huge change in your smile. Dental bonding is one example. We like to say the best kind of cosmetic dentistry we can do will give you the best value for the least amount of work. Cosmetic dentistry can be not only affordable but cost-effective.

With all dental procedures, it is your responsibility as the patient to fully investigate the dentist. Is he or she a member of the American Academy of Cosmetic Dentistry—more commonly known as the AACD? While it's not a prerequisite, this membership demonstrates that a dentist has a vested interest in the specialty, although not every AACD member is excellent at this craft.

The first thing you might ask a prospective cosmetic dentist is to show you some photographic examples of his or her work. Ask the dentist to put you in touch with others who have had work done. Good cosmetic dentists have stopping points throughout the procedure in order to determine whether they're meeting the patient's expectations—or are perhaps even going too far by assuming you want something changed that you don't. Again, the best cosmetic dentistry is the ***least invasive*** dentistry that gets you the results you want.

Cosmetic dentistry is something that shouldn't be sold. The dentist should be your "smile advisor" and say, "Okay, here's what we can do that can get you what you'd expect from your smile in the long run. You want white teeth that all are straight? Here's the least amount of dentistry we can do to get you there."

We are not magicians or superheroes (though sometimes we try to convince our children we are). We believe cosmetic dentistry's merits are limited only by the imagination. Its effects can be life-changing, as they were for Brian, Louise, Tiffany, Dixie, Tom, Ronald, Don, Pastor Terry, and so many others.

No matter what your dental history has been, it's worthwhile to get the best smile you can now. There is so much left in the world for each of us to accomplish.

Chapter 10

What to Expect from Us

And if not from us, then from another dentist

t may sound clichéd to say a "life of service" is what we aspire to, but it's absolutely true. At the very least, it's a large part of the goal that both of us set for ourselves a long time ago—maybe even in that Michigan high school where we first became friends.

We know that improving people's dental health can make a huge difference in their desire to move ahead and make valuable contributions in the world. More often than not, self-confidence includes appearance—or what we believe others see when they look at us. The odds are, people will lead more productive lives when they feel better about themselves.

In short, while we're not ministers or teachers, we want to use whatever talents and abilities we were given to enrich other people's lives. As a result of this philosophy, there's a lot you can expect from our practice. But first, we'd like you to know who we are.

Christian's story:

I was raised in a family where we were taught, emphatically, that in one way or another we were here to serve others. It was a mantra. My mother was a nurse and other relatives were also in the medical profession. For them, helping others was the purpose in life. My father was an architect, and even though he cringed at the sight of blood, he made clear by his example that blessing people carried great rewards.

I always knew I wanted to be my own boss. I left home at sixteen not because I didn't have terrific parents, but because my independence kept getting the better of me. Frankly, I considered starting a T-shirt company, because I had a propensity for building and creating (with Erector sets and Legos, for example) and expressing myself artistically, even though my business partner is the actual artist. At one point, although she recognized that I needed to make my own decisions, my mother was still able to exert some influence over me by questioning my career choice. Not that there's anything wrong with printing T-shirts—but I think she wondered just how that would help people. She was right.

A visit to my family dentist at the time proved discouraging—perhaps even frightening. "Don't go into dentistry," he'd warned me. "Dentistry is less than rewarding. It's grueling. The only reason I do it is to make a living."

It was clear that my own dentist wasn't happy, and I found it was most unsettling to know that someone with no interest in the profession had been working on our family's teeth! To be great at something, to provide the most benefit for those you treat, and to reap the highest personal rewards, you have to be passionate about it.

I met another dentist when I took an exploratory class in college to decide whether I was cut out for dentistry. My instructor told me how much he loved practicing dentistry, but he challenged me by saying he felt I wasn't sophisticated enough to be a good dentist. At the end of the course, he suggested I look into another field of work.

However, that "slap of the glove" only propelled me further in my resolve to enter the dentistry profession. Sure, his words stung—but only for about a minute. I'd given everything I had to that class, and I had really liked it, so I was determined not to stop there.

Both Joe and I took the test for admission to dental school at the same time and we both were accepted—with the added benefit that we could skip our senior year of college. It's rare that I've been without determination in my life, and the same goes for Joe, which has allowed us to build the Ballantyne Center for Dentistry into the celebrated, full-service adult dental practice it has become (more on that later).

Joe's story:

I grew up in a household where both my parents were medical professionals. My dad was a medical technologist and my mom a nurse. Though they never told me what career to choose, it was a foregone conclusion that I would be in the medical field in some capacity.

As a young child, I loved to tinker with things and had an artistic streak. I liked to play with acrylics, watercolors, and pencil drawings. At some point during grade school, I got the idea that I wanted to become a dentist. (And no, I didn't run around singing Herbie's song about wanting to be a dentist from the animated *Rudolph the Red-Nosed Reindeer*, though it occurred to me from time to time!)

My ACT college entrance exam scores weren't exceedingly high (more fuel for the increasingly popular belief that test scores are not indicative of one's ability and talents). In fact, at that time, a counselor told me I'd be lucky to become a garbage collector! How's that for helping the young people he was supposed to serve? My grades were fairly high, so I filed his inappropriate, highly destructive comments under "trash"— and like Christian, I rushed headlong toward my goal.

Though I was accepted into dental school, there was a question about whether I would make it through the program. Both my siblings had been awarded full scholarships as undergrads. They were high scholastic achievers, and nobody questioned whether they would be successful at whatever career they chose. But while I was an amiable young man with artistic talent, achieving high grades did not come easily for me. Even my father expressed his doubts that I'd make it all the way through dental school.

Christian has mentioned we were offered admission after our junior year of college, but mine didn't come about quite in the same way his did. During my application process and the first interview with the dean of admissions, I was advised to finish up an undergraduate degree and get "a bit more rounded experience" before reapplying to the dental school the following year. Perseverance was on my side that day. I told the dean that, though I respected his opinion, I would be getting into a dental school *this* year—and if not his school, there would be another dental school willing to accept my tuition payments.

It's all about perseverance at any age. I hope that's what I continue to impress upon my patients. If you want something badly enough, don't give up. Find someone who will listen, the way we do in our practice—someone who will get you on the path. When a patient has been told by another dentist that something can't be done, we usually question why. It may require some rethinking and retooling of the original goal, but often we find a way to make it happen.

We've both been challenged in our lives in various ways. We've lived it, and because of that, we can empathize with our patients.

Out on our own

While we came to North Carolina separately, we ended up working together in a group practice owned by an insurance company. We were given a little more *carte blanche* than many dentists in the same circumstances, so we were fine there for a while, but we knew we had to leave eventually. The company policies changed. The owners had begun to mandate that we see more and more people, carry out procedures in the least expensive way possible, use cheaper materials, and cut lab costs—just to improve the bottom line, with no attention to quality. The new emphasis on profitability made it clear that this group no longer had the patients' best interests in mind. At that point, we decided to unleash our own vision and build the dental practice of our dreams.

In **Coriolanus**, Shakespeare said, "The people are the city." That's exactly how we feel about a dental practice: The people are the practice. We couldn't endorse compromise, so we launched our own company: the Ballantyne Center for Dentistry.

Practicing ethics and values

We'd like you to know about our philosophy and also what you should expect from any dentist who, like us, wants to provide the best experience and solutions for their patients. We'd like to talk about how our practice operates. These are ideas we proudly share with other dentists who are earnestly changing the landscape of adult dentistry.

You know from previous chapters that our focus is on Baby Boomers, and within that demographic, we also treat patients with whom other dentists are not comfortable, for one reason or another. We treat people who fear going to the dentist and people with compound problems whose mouths have been improperly treated by other dentists, and more. Because we see each patient as a whole—rather than just going "tooth by tooth"—we have learned to focus on the big picture.

We armed ourselves with as much advanced education as possible in adult treatments and procedures. We've said before that, when all you have is a hammer, everything looks like a nail. This has provided the kind of incentive we've needed to study a broad range of services, resulting in a larger set of "tools" and providing a wealth of options for our patients.

Often, patients come to us with an idea that they want veneers, for example. They may not have a clear idea of what exactly veneers are or know whether they are good candidates for the procedure. What they really mean is they want a healthy, straight, white, beautiful smile. There are so many different ways to attain this goal—including veneers, dental implants, and other options and combinations under the headings of cosmetic and restorative dentistry—and we believe people should have the advantage of having all these options under one roof, whenever possible. That's our objective. State-of-the-art equipment, technology, pain management, sedation, and certainly clinician education and experience are all paramount to making this happen.

Here's a good analogy. If your child was spending a considerable amount of time anywhere but at home, possibly viewing things on the Internet at various neighbors' homes over which you had no control because you could not be there 24/7, how would you solve the problem? Move away? That's a possibility, but it's a gigantic, time-consuming, and costly inconvenience, unless you were planning to move anyway—and it might take months or years to find another place and sell yours. Rather than an upheaval like that, why not make your home *the* place to be—the best destination house on the block? What could you do to make your home the place all the kids wanted to be?

Christian was actually in this situation. He put in a swimming pool, creating a kids' entertainment space with both recreational and Internet options indoors for inclement weather—but which could be overseen and controlled by a competent adult.

We have applied this lesson to our practice. We have enough treatment options under one roof (sorry—no pool!) to draw people to enjoy coming to our office. We provide dozens of ideas and treatment plans to solve almost any dental problem.

Interestingly, when the contractor came to Christian's house to discuss installing a pool, he asked what he should do—what the plan was for the project. The request was curious, because it was almost like the dentist asking the patient what should be done. But upon further discussion, the contractor revealed that most people automatically tell him what they want—just like the patient coming in with a request for veneers, without really knowing what else is out there that may work better or differently.

Wouldn't it make more sense to describe what *experience* you want when you walk outside to go to the pool and what *feelings* it should create in you as you enjoy it? In the case of the contractor or the dentist, it's then incumbent upon the expert involved to listen carefully to the goals you have in mind, and then to suggest the best way to get there or propose alternatives that might even work better. Who knows? They may surprise you with the kind of solution they can provide!

Starting with the questions

In our practice, we start with a lot of questions that help us determine your needs and desires, your ideas and budget. Do you want white, straight teeth? Teeth with which you can chew steak or raw vegetables? Do you want a smile that gets everyone's attention? Do you just want to have the confidence to know, when you interact with friends, colleagues, or family, that they are focused on you and not your teeth? Tell us what your priorities are, and what the experience should be for you— what the big picture is—and we'll tell you how many ways there are to get there. We'll provide a lot of options. It might mean a root canal and crown on tooth number eleven, an implant next to it, and four veneers on top. Dentistry is definitely **not** one-size-fits-all.

It's important to keep in mind that dentistry is about emotion. You want to be happy—even if concealing your teeth, shying away from family, work, and social engagements, or living with pain and forgoing favorite foods has become the norm for you. You might not remember what it was like *not* to live with shame and feel bad about yourself.

You want your confidence back. You want to be able to kiss your wife at the end of the day and not have her pull back because she is sickened by your breath or the condition of your teeth. Perhaps you want to go out again, feel attractive, and experience a new relationship, because you are starting over. Maybe you want to be the star of the show at public speaking engagements in your future.

Instead of coming in and asking for a partial, or a bridge, or veneers, we'd like to hear about the big picture—your immediate and long-term goals for how you'd like to *feel*—so we can determine how best to help you get there.

Creative dentistry is not cookie-cutter dentistry. It's not about across-the-board solutions. It's about listening and customizing your dental plan. In some practices—especially those that are driven by insurance or corporate practices, such as those referenced in Chapter 6—the patient goes in requesting a specific procedure. The dentist tells them whether or not they can do it. There aren't a lot of options offered.

In other practices, the patient is told, "Okay, and this is how I'm going to do it," and the patient, with no knowledge of other options, agrees. Anyone who questions the dentist's recommendations, or is looking for some flexibility in the treatment plan, might be sent elsewhere, leaving the patient frustrated or bewildered.

We believe that no matter what you want, or what we suggest, there are different paths to get there. We try to provide the "value engineering" we talked about earlier, meaning we try to find the option that fits your budget and lifestyle. How can you get to the finish line—not necessarily in the least expensive way, but in a way that provides the most value for the money you are spending? And in deciding on a treatment plan, how can you take advantage of any insurance benefits that may be available to you?

At the beginning of this chapter, we talked about how we chose a profession that lets us serve people. When people think of a life of service, they might think about ministry, teaching, medicine, or public office. Few people consider dentistry as a service profession—but for us, and for other dentists who think as we do, it clearly is.

Insurance companies and the corporate mentality have infiltrated our profession in recent years, which has made dentistry more convenient for some patients but has left others feeling lost. We have adopted the new model that is emerging in dentistry, and we are hopeful that in it, you will find solutions to your problems. Again, we are not the only ones breaking new ground here. Adult dentistry is evolving from the way it was twenty or thirty years ago. Dentists all over the world are recognizing that fact and acting on it. We are proud to count ourselves among the members of that highly dedicated group.

Chapter 11

Ready for the New Patient Experience

Are we made for each other?

I f we could design our ideal patient, it might be you! Throughout the book, we've talked about how our practice focuses on the 1946-1964 Baby Boom generation—individuals ages fifty-three to seventy-one and older—and how important it is for people to be aware that dentistry isn't what it was fifteen or twenty years ago. There is a whole new world of options and bigger, better, brighter results. The right patient-dentist fit is integral to making that happen.

Dentistry has become sub-specialized. Specialties used to be more rigid and traditional—dental care was all about the orthodontist, the endodontist, the periodontist, and the like. If you didn't need a specialist in one of those categories, you went to the general/family dentist.

Today, it's very different. The family dentist may no longer be the best choice for older adults. There's a difference between family dentistry and adult dentistry. We hope our patients understand this going in and are open to this reality.

In our adult dentistry practice, we focus on cosmetic, restoration, and implant procedures. If you are a Baby Boomer, you may have missing teeth or teeth that are starting to wear down, presenting functional challenges and aesthetic issues. Perhaps you wear dentures that are uncomfortable, a hindrance, and/or are worn and cracked. You may have had a series of mediocre or bad experiences with dentists along the way. Maybe you feel—as Jack Nicholson famously said in the film ***Terms of Endearment***—that you would "rather stick needles in (your) eyes" than go through another dental appointment. But you will find that becoming our patient can be infinitely less painful and happily rewarding!

The "perfect" cosmetic smile

Realistic expectations are important. While we do our utmost to make sure you have everything you want for a fabulous, functional smile, you won't necessarily find our patients in the pages of *Variety* or *The Hollywood Reporter*. If your goal is "Chiclet-white" teeth lined up like a picket fence, we may not be the best choice for you. Though we strive for the best results, we don't promote "perfection" when it comes to esthetics. We know that perfect doesn't look great—in fact, perfect looks *fake*.

You know when you see someone smile and you can tell right away that they've had something done to their teeth? That's what we are talking about. A healthy, optimally functioning, natural-looking mouth is our goal. It's realistic, and it can be stunning if it displays uniformity and cleanliness. If done properly, when you smile, people will only be impressed with how fantastic your smile looks. If that aligns with the goals you have for your own smile, we might be an excellent fit.

We know money counts!

We want to make our services accessible to adults who desire them. That means it's important to us to come up with individualized treatment plans that work within our patients' budgets. In fact, one of the biggest factors that keep people from coming to the dentist for extensive dental work is cost. In today's world, we know we have to be flexible and provide a number of payment plans and options for our patients when it comes to finances. We like to say we specialize in helping people afford dentistry. But results can cost money.

If you don't have enough disposable income, you may have to be flexible and willing to sacrifice or postpone a new car, vacation, home renovation, or something equally important. But prioritizing is part of what we all do as adults. If you are willing, we are able!

Going off to dreamland ... safely

In our practice, we offer many different ways to have the most pleasant and relaxed dental office experience. Sedation has become tremendously popular in the last decade, and there are many different forms and ways to achieve this for our patients. These methods range from nitrous oxide (also called "laughing gas") to an oral sedative, I.V. sedation, and even general anesthesia. But it is important for you to know the pros and cons, safety, and limitations of each of these systems. We believe that if you know what to expect, you will have the best experience, so we educate our patients about what these expectations should be.

In Chapter 2, we recounted the tale of Christian flying over his bicycle's handlebars and the painful, unacceptable treatment he received afterward. Because of that experience, he is a ***bona fide*** dental phobic. We hope sharing that story underscored our sensitivity to the problem. Our goal is to help remove any fear you may have acquired from negative past experiences, replacing it with empathy, compassion, and a customized treatment plan just for you. This, in turn, builds up your trust and confidence, producing outstanding results.

Healthy ideals

We find it empowering to work with patients who put their health at the top of their agendas. Chapter 4, which explains how good overall health is connected with good oral health, is important on many fronts. From a patient-dentist relationship aspect, it means you will care about yourself enough to do what is necessary at home to maintain the dental work we've completed, along with scheduled cleanings and check-ups.

From a dentist-patient relationship perspective, it means we know you are serious about our efforts, which are the sum total of years and years of continuing education, hard work, increasing expertise, training in new technology, efficient work flow, and so much more. We make a considerable investment in you, and we know you will protect that investment, just as a museum maintains a fine painting. While no one is perfect, and mishaps surely occur, we are always here to help you. We feel good knowing you are making the effort to preserve what we've accomplished for you.

Many of our patients come to us in physical and/or emotional pain. The condition of their mouths has created problems that range from precluding a healthy diet to holding them back from professional success to stopping them from socializing with friends and coworkers. For people like Louise (Chapter 4), even participating socially with their families is impossible, because of the way they feel about their oral health.

We've shared with you the stories of patients like Brian at the car dealership (Chapter 1), whose professional—and personal—life was transformed when his teeth were repaired. Tiffany and Pastor Terry (both in Chapter 9) are shining examples of the redemptive—yes, redemptive!—power of quality dentistry. If you need this kind of life change, we are here to help.

We certainly don't want people to experience pain of any kind, but we recognize that emotional or physical pain can be the catalyst for seeking help. A patient in pain often feels ready to take action, and we like that attitude. They want to move forward, get out of pain, and change their lives. We are able to jump in and help them.

Clearly, not all patients visit our office with their lives in crisis—but if they do, we embrace the chance to help them with a treatment plan that moves as quickly as possible, taking their circumstances into account.

What we do

We treat dental conditions, such as gum disease, missing teeth, tooth sensitivity, dry mouth, tooth decay, worn-out fillings, worn-down teeth, and bad breath, to name a few. We screen for oral cancer, fix broken teeth, address the causes of mouth sores, treat tooth erosion, address acid problems, and create long-lasting, beautiful smiles—and so much more.

We like to say that, to us, you are not just a set of teeth. You are an individual with your own short- and long-term goals and objectives, your own lifestyle, unique experiences, and financial plans. If you are willing to be forthcoming in telling us your story so we can best determine if you fit our patient profile—and if we believe we can meet all of your needs—you are likely a great candidate for Ballantyne Center for Dentistry.

It's your turn!

Thank you for reading our book. If you've gotten to this point, consider yourself fully equipped to find the right dentist. You are ready to take action toward a healthier mouth and more spectacular smile, and you are now informed enough to ask for a variety of options to get there. If you think you're a good candidate for our practice, we'd like to get to know you and help you move confidently toward your goal.

Please go immediately to www.ballantynedentistry.com or www.charlottedentalimplant.com and take the next step with us. Welcome!

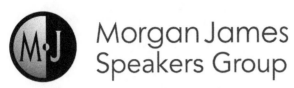

Morgan James
Speakers Group

We connect Morgan James published
authors with live and online events
and audiences who will benefit
from their expertise.

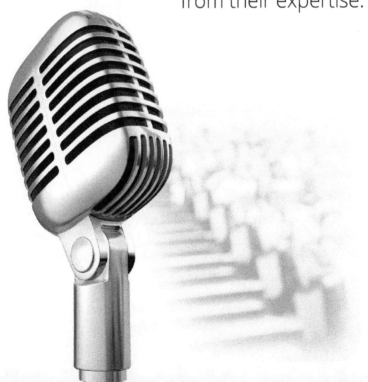